W9-CZU-344

THE COMPLETE IDIOT'S GUIDE™ TO

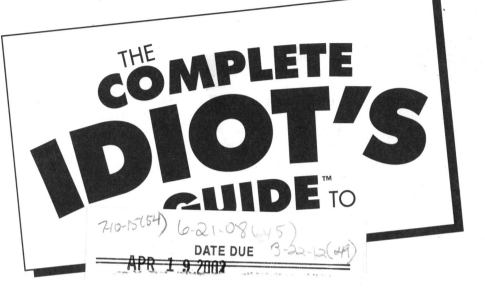

Healthy Stretching

by Chris Verna and Steve Hosid

alpha books

A Division of Macmillan General Reference
A Simon & Schuster Macmillan Company
1633 Broadway, New York, NY 10019

THE COMPLETE IDIOT'S GUIDE name and design are trademarks of Macmillan, Inc.

International Standard Book Number: 0-02-862127-1
Library of Congress Catalog Card Number: 97-80934

00 99 98   8 7 6 5 4 3 2

Interpretation of the printing code: the rightmost number of the first series of numbers is the year of the book's printing; the rightmost number of the second series of numbers is the number of the book's printing. For example, a printing code of 98-1 shows that the first printing occurred in 1998.

Printed in the United States of America

This publication contains information based on the research and experience of its author and is designed to provide useful advice with regard to the subject matter covered. The author and publishers are not engaged in rendering medical or other professional services in this publication. Circumstances vary for practitioners of the activities covered herein, and this publication should not be used without prior consultation from a competent medical professional.

The author and publisher expressly disclaim any responsibility for any liability, loss, injury, or risk, personal or otherwise, which is incurred as a consequence, directly or indirectly, of the use and application of any of the contents of this book.

Brand Manager
Kathy Nebenhaus

Executive Editor
Gary M. Krebs

Managing Editor
Bob Shuman

Senior Editor
Nancy Mikhail

Development Editor
Joan Paterson

Production Editor
Lynn Northrup

Technical Editor
Chris Verna

Editorial Assistant
Maureen Horn

Cover Designer
Michael Freeland

Cartoonist
Judd Winick

Photos
Steve Hosid

Designer
Glenn Larsen

Indexer
Chris Barrick

Production Team
Angela Calvert, Pamela Woolf

Demonstrators
*Chris Verna, Lisa Kopplin, Jackie Gramkow
Ellen, Adam, and Jordan Stokey; Carolyn Boublis*

Primary Photo Location
Arnold Palmer's Bay Hill Club and Lodge, Orlando, Florida

Anatomy Artist and Photo Coordinator
Jill Ashton Hosid

Contents at a Glance

Part 1: Understanding Stretching and Flexibility   **1**

  1   Here's Looking at You, Kid—Your Flexibility Self-Test   3
Mr. Stretch helps evaluate your flexibility. We have to start somewhere.

  2   Tell Me a Little About Yourself!   21
Your lifestyle and history—how they affect your flexibility.

  3   Your Body's Political System and How it Should Work Together   33
Here's how it's supposed to work. Maybe you need a re-call election.

  4   Okay Gang, Here's What Stretching Will Do for You   43
Mr. Stretch puts you on the road to flexibility and feeling better.

Part 2: Stretch the Day: Mr. Stretch's Pick-and-Choose Menu   **51**

  5   Good Morning: The Wake-Up Wonders   53
Starting your day with a flexible smile.

  6   Mid-Afternoon Energy Boosters   73
Keep perky with these quick healthy stretches. Fewer calories and more energy than a candy bar.

  7   Nightcaps: To Be Shared With Another   91
Can you think of a better way to end the day?

Part 3: Stretching for Real-Life Situations   **109**

  8   Sitters of the World Unite: Get Vacationing Muscles Back to Work   111
Stiff necks and sore wrists take a leave of absence as you reboot your body.

  9   Physical Professions or Hobbies: Stiffness, Stiffness Everywhere   123
If you lift, pound, bend, or climb, Mr. Stretch has some good stretches for you.

  10   Captured Commuters   139
Stuck at 30,000 feet or in rush-hour traffic? Try these.

Part 4: Good Sports: Mr. Stretch's Program for Flexibility   **153**

  11   Golf: Rotating All the Way to the Hole   155
With clients winning nine major titles, Mr. Stretch has a program for you.

12 Tennis: Love the Flexibility 165
You'll love the stretching approach to better tennis.

13 Leg Sports: Walking, Rollerblading, Cycling, Running, and Climbing 177
Since you like to move, you'll love these lubricating stretches.

14 Swimming: Fluidity in the Water 189
Different strokes for different folks...and stretches to match.

15 Skiing and Other Winter Sports: Cold-Weather Engine Protection 197
With these stretches you'll never be left out in the cold.

Part 5: Special Situations Require Special Stretches 207

16 Pregnancy Stretching: Expecting to Be Flexible 209
Some gentle stretches for the changes in your life. Partners welcome.

17 Let's Stretch the Kids: Flexibility for Life 219
Quality time as a flexibility-conscious parent.

18 Senior Flexibility: Healthy Stretching for an Active Lifestyle 231
Stay flexible and enjoy an active lifestyle.

Part 6: Mr. Stretch's Program for Improving the Quality of Your Life With Stretching 243

19 Healthy Stretching Your Feet, Ankles, and Calves 245
A variety of stretches to help develop and maintain joint flexibility.

20 Healthy Stretching Your Knees, Hips, and Hamstrings 255
Stretches to help you maintain an active lifestyle.

21 Healthy Stretching Your Back and Abdomen 273
Maintaining flexibility to keep you off your back.

22 Healthy Stretching Your Shoulders and Neck 285
Mr. Stretch's exercises for less tension and more flexibility.

23 Healthy Stretching Your Elbows and Wrists 295
Stretches to help keep your arms and wrists flexible.

Glossary 303
Have a question about what something means? Check Mr. Stretch's stretching-related definitions.

Index 305

Contents

Part 1: Understanding Stretching and Flexibility — 1

1 Here's Looking at You, Kid—Your Flexibility Self-Test — 3

Who's Walking in Your Footsteps? 4
Waddling Duck 5
Lost Pigeon 5
If Your Posture Could Speak 6
The Statue of Liberty 6
Leaning Tower of Pisa 9
How Do You Look From the Side? 10
Knees and Ankles, the Propellers 11
Getting a Knee Up 11
Knee Differential Test 12
Ankles Away 13
Okay, You're Not Elvis, But How Flexible Are
Your Hips? 13
Shoulders—You've Been Carrying the World on Them 14
Elbows and Wrists 16
Are You an Elbow Bender? 16
Do Your Wrists Have Trouble Waving Goodbye? 17
Sticking Your Neck Out 18
The Physical Part of the Test Is Over 19
The Least You Need to Know 19

2 Tell Me a Little About Yourself! — 21

Are You a Sitter? 22
Are You a Stander? 23
Have You Ever Been Injured? 23
Bone Fractures 23
Muscle Strains 24
Ligament Strains 24
Be Honest Now...How Are You Built? 24
NFL Lineman 25
Marathon Runner 25
Workout Woman 25
Supermodel 26
Do I Really Have to Tell You, Mr. Stretch? 26

Tell Me How You Play! 26
Endurance Sports 26
Aerobic Sports 27
Weekend Warrior 28
I Get a Round In! 28
Well, Mr. Stretch, I Have This Great Couch! 29
I'm Not Your Mom, But Where Does it Hurt? 29
I Have This Pain in My Neck 29
Can I Exchange This Back for One That Works? 30
I Love Standing for Five Hours on Cross-Country
Flights! 30
Is That Your Knees or Pipes Creaking? 30
I'd Like to Sue This Ankle for Non-Support! 30
How Do the French Say "Everywhere"? 31
The Least You Need to Know 31

3 Your Body's Political System: How it Should Work Together 33

The Constitution of Flexibility 34
Bones: The Executive Branch 34
Muscles: The Legislative Branch 35
Joints: The Judiciary 37
If Your Body Is a Computer, Some Muscles May
Have a "Virus" 40
Compensating for the Vacationing Muscle 40
Healthy Stretching Sends the Muscle a Wake-Up Call ... 41
The Least You Need to Know 41

4 Okay, Gang, Here's What Healthy Stretching Will Do for You 43

Together We've Identified Your Problems 45
If You're Having Pain, You Should See a Doctor 45
So, Mr. Stretch, How Do I Start? 45
Blend Healthy Stretching With Other Exercise
Programs 46
You're Almost Ready to Start: Some More
Important Tips 47
The 15-Second Hold: 15 Seconds That Can Change
Your Life 47
The Squeaking Wheel Gets More Grease 48

Connect Your Stretches: Several Areas May Need to Be
Re-Educated 49
The Least You Need to Know 49

**Part 2: Stretch the Day: Mr. Stretch's
Pick-and-Choose Menu**   **51**

5 Good Morning: The Wake-Up Wonders   **53**

Yawn Busters—Not Even Out of Bed and You're
Already Stretching 54
    Undercover Body Stretch 54
    Morning Hamstring Stretch 54
    Two Knees to the Chin 56
    Two Knees to the Side 56
Mr. Stretch's Healthy Way to Get Out of Bed 57
The Floor Four: Learning From Your Dog or Cat 58
    Back Arch 58
    Praying Stretch 59
    Torso Press Up 60
    Walking Wake-Up Stretch 61
The Facial Two 62
    Neck Toner 62
    Chin Chin 63
Morning Power: After-Your-Shower Stimulators 64
    Front Bend 64
    Bend Over Twist 66
    Landing Eagle 66
    Wall Side Bend 68
Towel Time: Don't Hang it Up to Dry Just Yet 69
    Towel-Free Stretch 69
    Horizontal Towel Stretch 70
    Vertical Towel Stretch 71
The Least You Need to Know 71

6 Mid-Afternoon Energy Boosters   **73**

Your Energy Foundation 74
    Front Squat 74
    Frog Squat 75
    Squat Lunge 76

Standing Calf Stretch 77
Front Hip Flexor 77
Energy Enhancers 78
Hands Up 78
Side Bend 78
Squat and Sit 80
Afternoon Squat and Twist 81
Tension Relaxers 82
Shoulder Shrug 83
Seated Rowing Motion 84
Overhead Shrug 85
Shoulder Twist 86
Neck Minders 86
Head Forward and Back Stretch 87
Ear to Shoulder 88
Head Rotation 89
The Least You Need to Know 90

7 Nightcaps: To Be Shared With Another   91

Back to Backs 92
Extended Back Stretcher 92
Extended Side to Side 94
Suite Treats 95
Back Rockers 95
Seated Shoulder Stretchers 96
Togetherness Side-to-Side Stretches 97
One-Arm Twist 98
Hip Huggers 99
Seated Back Stretchers 99
Sitting Twist 100
Two for One 100
Nighttime Knee Bender 101
Leg-Lifter, Two-Step Stretch 102
Side Quad Stretch 103
Diamond Stretch 104
Last-Call Stretches 105
Soothing Gentle Back Stretch 105
Rotating Rhythm Stretch 106
Curtain Call Stretch 107
The Least You Need to Know 107

Part 3: Stretching for Real-Life Situations   **109**

8 Sitters of the World Unite! Get Vacationing Muscles Back to Work   **111**

It's Not Always the Boss Giving You That Pain
  in the Neck 112
    Tension Deleter 112
    One More Neck Stretch 113
Carpal Tunnel Syndrome: Curse of the Keyboard 113
    Your Mouse Gets Better Care Than You Do 114
    Backhand Push 114
    Wrist Relievers 115
Re-Educating Your Sitting Muscles 116
    Sitting Hip Stretch 116
    Sitting Outside Hip Stretch 117
    Quad Muscle Wake-Up 118
    Leg Stretch 119
    Hamstring Standing Stretch 120
Reboot Your Body 121
    Programmer Stretch 1 121
    Programmer Stretch 2 122
The Least You Need to Know 122

9 Physical Professions or Hobbies: Stiffness, Stiffness Everywhere   **123**

Compared to You, Million-Dollar Athletes Have
  it Easy 124
Lifters: Mr. Stretch Helps You Carry the Load 125
    Lower Body Standing Stretch 125
    Hamstring Conditioner 126
    Standing Quad Conditioner 127
    Inner-Thigh Conditioner 127
Arm Benders: Join Mr. Stretch at the Bar 129
    One-Armer Stretch 129
    Double-Handed Stretch 130
    Backward Arm Conditioner 131
Benders: Mr. Stretch Plants the Seeds for Healthy
  Stretching 132
    Back Planter 132
    Both Sides Body Conditioner 134
    Hamstring Planter 134

Stop the Presses! Mr. Stretch Shows Backache to
    Be a Thing of the Past 136
        Pipe Bender Stretch 136
        Pipe Twister Stretch 138
    The Least You Need to Know 138

10 Captured Commuters   139

    Ode to the Captured Commuter 139
    The 30,000-Feet Energy Secret 139
    A 45-Million-Dollar Stretching Machine 140
        The Fighter Pilot Stretch 141
        Flaps-Up Arm Stretch 141
        Banking Rotation 142
        Landing Gear Neck Stretch 142
        Serving-Tray, Shoulder-Blade Stretch 144
        Tail-Section Stretch 144
        Landing Gear Up 146
    Highway Prisoners 147
        Steering-Wheel Twist 147
        Door Stretch 148
        Head-Rest Arm Stretch 149
        One-Arm Seat Stretch 150
        Lumbar Roll Stretch 150
        Accelerator Stretch 151
    Mr. Stretch Knows Best 152
    The Least You Need to Know 152

**Part 4: Good Sports: Mr. Stretch's Program
            for Flexibility   153**

11 Golf: Rotating All the Way to the Hole   155

    Rotational Golf 156
    Golf Carts: More Than Transportation Around
        the Course 157
        Cart Quad Stretch 157
        Birdie Hip Stretch 158
        Eagle Inner Thigh Stretch 159
        Long Driver Shoulder Turn 160
    Address for Success 162
    Stretch for a Rotational Swing.................................... 163
    The Least You Need to Know 163

12 Tennis: Love the Flexibility   **165**

The Weekend Warrior Syndrome 166
Upper Body Stretches: Stretching From the Top Down 167
     Behind the Back Racket Stretch 167
     Under Grip Net Stretch 168
     Avoid Tennis Elbow: Over Grip Net Stretch 169
Serving Stretches 170
     First Serve Stretch 170
     Biceps Fence Stretcher 171
Legs: The Power of the Game 172
     Ankle Stretcher 172
     Standing Quad Stretch 173
     Bench Stretch Your Hamstring 174
Sliding Stretches 175
The Least You Need to Know 176

13 Leg Sports: Walking, Rollerblading, Cycling, Running, and Climbing   **177**

How the Natural Runners Stretch 178
What Can Go Wrong 179
     Runners: Pounding Away 179
     Cyclists: Seated Rotational Movers 179
     Rollerbladers: Pushing-Off Hip Alert 179
     Climbing Machines: Stairways to Tightness 180
Weekend Warriors: The Vicious Cycle of Inflexibility 180
Mr. Stretch's Flexibility Favorites 180
     Calves Pole Stretch 180
     Hamstring Striding Stretch 182
     Dynamic Quad Stretch 183
     Inner Thigh Straddle Stretch 184
     Standing Hip Stretch 185
     Kneeling Shin Stretch 186
     One-Legged Climber Stretch 187
The Least You Need to Know 188

14 Swimming: Fluidity in the Water   **189**

Swimming Muscle Harmony 190
The Water Ballet of the Joints 190
Tuning Up the Engine Stretches 192

Sleeper Stretch 193

Freestyle Stretch 194

Lower Body Power Stretches 195

Shin Splits Stretch 195

The Frog 196

The Least You Need to Know 196

15 Skiing and Other Winter Sports: Cold-Weather Engine Protection   197

Body Awareness 198

Healthy Stretching Improves Body Awareness 199

Asking Santa for Flexibility Doesn't Quite Make it 199

Fall-Line Favorites 199

Edge Sharpener 200

Shock Absorber 202

Mogul Tamers 203

Skiers' Quad Stretch 203

Skiers' Standing-Hip Stretch 204

Black Diamond Stretch 205

Top of the Run Stretch 206

The Least You Need to Know 206

Part 5: Special Situations Require Special Stretches 207

16 Pregnancy Stretching: Expecting to Be Flexible   209

Healthy Stretching During Pregnancy 210

Three "M" Stretches: Making Mom Merry 210

Back Bend-Over 210

Standing Shoulder Twist 211

Crossover Stretch 212

Adjusting as You Adjust 212

Knee-Neck Stretch 213

Side Quad Stretch 214

Two-Legged Pelvic Raise 215

Hamstring Stretch 216

Let a Partner Help 216

Partner Side Stretch 217

Partner Hip Stretch 218

The Least You Need to Know 218

17 Let's Stretch the Kids: Flexibility for Life   **219**

My Flexibility Problems as a Kid 219
Be a Flexibility-Conscious Parent 220
Children Are Sitters Too! 220
How to Start—Become Mr. Stretch's Assistant Coach 221
Fun Favorites 221
    One-Foot Stretch 222
    Feeling Taller 222
    Hands Above the Head Stretch 223
    Soccer Stretch 223
    Side Stretch 224
    Cannon Ball 225
    Back Leaner 226
    Hamstring Stretch 227
    Campfire Sitting Stretch 228
    Swordsmen Lunge 229
Neck Stretches 230
The Least You Need to Know 230

**18 Senior Flexibility: Healthy Stretching for an
Active Lifestyle**   **231**

How Healthy Stretching Helped Carolyn 232
Mr. Stretch, Can Healthy Stretching Help Me Too? 233
Senior Savvy Stretches 233
    Overhead Side Stretch 234
    Standing Shoulder Twist 235
    Cross-Body Arm Stretch 236
The "Flexibility Five" Stretches 237
    En Garde 237
    Side Lunge 238
    Senior Hamstring Stretch 238
    Senior Modified Pretzel 240
    Senior Side-Quad Stretch 241
The Least You Need to Know 242

Part 6: Mr. Stretch's Program for Improving the Quality of Your Life With Stretching 243

19 Healthy Stretching Your Feet, Ankles, and Calves 245

Standing Calf Stretch 246
Level 2 Standing Heel and Calf Stretch 248
Level 3 Heel and Calf Stretch 249
Shin Splint Stretch 250
Outside of Ankle Stretch 251
Toe and Foot Stretch 252
Ankle Rotation 253
The Least You Need to Know 254

20 Healthy Stretching Your Knees, Hips, and Hamstrings 255

Pretzel Stretch 256
Modified Pretzel Stretch 257
Full Pretzel Stretch 258
Seated Hip Stretch 260
Standing Inner Thigh Stretch 262
Frog Stretch 263
One-Legged Frog Stretch 264
Level 1 Triangle Quad Stretch 265
Advanced Triangle Quad Stretch 266
Chair Lunge 267
Hamstring Stretch 267
Level 1 Hamstring Stretch 268
Level 2 Hamstring Stretch 269
Level 3 Hamstring Stretch 270
Butterfly Stretch 271
The Least You Need to Know 271

21 Healthy Stretching Your Back and Abdomen 273

One Knee to Chest 275
Two Knees to Chest 276
Sitting Lower Back Stretch 277
Shoulder Back Roll 278
Torso Stretch 279
Level 1 Two Knees Over 280
Levels 2 and 3 One Knee Over 281

Side Overhead Arch 282
The Least You Need to Know 283

22 Healthy Stretching Your Shoulders and Neck   285

Level 1 Neck Side-to-Side Stretch 286
Level 2 Seated Neck Stretch 287
Level 3 Back Neck Stretch 288
Chin-Ups Stretch 289
Shoulder Arm Across the Body Stretch 290
Biceps Stretch 290
Triceps Stretch 291
Sleeper Stretch 292
The Least You Need to Know 293

23 Healthy Stretching Your Elbows and Wrists   295

Straight Elbow Stretch 296
Table Elbow Stretch 297
Pointed Elbow Stretch 297
Wrist Twist Stretch Down 298
Wrist and Elbow Stretch 299
Pushing Wrist Stretches 300
Side Wrist Stretches 301
The Least You Need to Know 302

Glossary   303

Index   305

Foreword

I wish Chris lived next door. There's no doubt I have developed more body awareness as a result of Chris Verna's healthy stretching program. Once you realize how it feels when your body is in the right positions, you do almost anything to keep it that way. I now know when my leg is not planting correctly or when my elbow and shoulder are not in the correct position to deliver the pitch with maximum velocity.

I met Chris Verna at a point in my career where the baseball season was really taking a toll on me physically. Then my agent, Myles Shoda, told me what Chris had accomplished with some of his clients. I met with Chris, who introduced his healthy stretching program and explained what he wanted to do.

One of my problems was a shoulder that separated from time to time. We all tend to think that if we have a pain in the shoulder, it must be caused by the shoulder; a pain in the hip must originate in the hip. Chris put me on a stretching program that helped me understand how the body works and saved me from shoulder surgery. My shoulder today is probably 30 times stronger than it was.

If I hadn't started working with Chris, I would have missed a lot of action. Our team's orthopedic surgeon has been amazed at the results. If you play my sport as long as I have, you get accustomed to the way things feel. And you fight a war to maintain them. Chris's healthy stretching program allowed me to free up certain parts of my body. As a pitcher, I throw about 130 pitches each game. The concern will normally be with your arm and shoulder. People don't realize that a pitcher also has to pick up his leg 130 times, and if you can do that more easily, everything works better together. I'm fortunate to have two of baseball's best trainers with the Braves who treat me on a daily basis. But, away from the field, Chris helps me work on areas that I need to concentrate on.

Stretching with Chris during the first off-season resulted in a spring training where it was obvious I could throw harder and faster. Chris's technique of healthy stretching works perfectly for me. His program allows me to extend and stay stronger. That really shows up in the playoffs, where I have to pitch with only three days' rest in between starts. Chris and his program have allowed more of my talents to shine on a continual basis.

When you're young, you think you don't need to stretch. This is a concern for parents and their children. I developed a very nasty groin injury dating back to high school that showed up every year at some point until stretching with Chris's program helped my body change.

Chris has helped me a tremendous amount in my career. I know healthy stretching will improve your body awareness and your athletic ability, and help prevent injury and reduce the stress that accumulates in your muscles.

John Smoltz
1996 Cy Young Award-winning pitcher with the Atlanta Braves

Introduction

Mention the word "stretching" a few centuries ago and absolute terror would set in. The stretching rack was a favorite play toy of Torquemada, the Spanish Inquisition's Grand Inquisitor. Improved athletic ability and a stress-reduced lifestyle were hardly primary concerns. Along those same lines, getting your neck stretched became unpopular in America's Wild West. While not especially time-consuming, it did interrupt an active lifestyle. Of course, not much equipment was needed—just a horse, a rope, a tree, and you!

In today's contemporary world, successful athletes follow a conditioning program that includes stretching. Professional athletes compete at incredibly high levels of proficiency. Golfers drive the ball farther then ever, tennis players serve at 100 mph-plus, runners are constantly setting new world records. Equipment is a big reason and the singular most important piece of equipment is the athlete's own body. As a plus factor, correct stretching also cuts down on the risk of a sports-related injury. These same principles apply to any person with an active lifestyle.

I work with many of the world's top athletes as their flexibility specialist. Now, for 24 hours a day, I am going to work with you in the pages of this Guide. I'm not going to preach to you about a healthy lifestyle, losing weight, or joining a health club. In fact, you don't need to buy anything or dress in special clothes. You already have everything you need. I'm ready to start working along with you whenever you want to begin.

What You'll Find in This Book

I hope you'll find that healthy stretching is not time-consuming and blends in with your lifestyle. In fact, the photos we use to guide you along were shot right in the very same type of locations you may find yourself in. You can be confident that we'll guide you every step of the way as you do the healthy stretches. It's important to feel I'm right there with you, making sure you're doing the stretches correctly. Healthy stretching does not mean painful, quick movements. Instead it's a way of gently saying to your muscles, "I'm going to help you, so that you can help me."

The Guide is divided into six parts. Part 1 begins in the same way it would if you came to my Chris Verna Training Center in Boca Raton, Florida. I'll guide you through a flexibility self-test. It's very simple and together we can see where some of your flexibility problems are. Chapter 2 will help us learn more about your lifestyle and the effect it may be having on your flexibility. Chapters 3 and 4 explain why you'll feel better as you do the healthy stretches, along with some unique information on how your body works.

Part 2 features healthy stretches you can do all day long, beginning before you get out of bed. You'll find a chapter on stretches you can do with a partner, before bedtime. Part 3 goes right to your daily lifestyle. If you work in an office, have a physical profession, or are ever stuck in your car or in a plane as a Captured Commuter, you'll find some healthy stretches to help you stay flexible and feel better.

Part 4 is where you can find the sports chapters and I'll show you how to get the most from your body, just as I do with the champion athletes I work with. Part 5 features special situations where healthy stretching can help—during pregnancy, with your family, and during the senior years. Finally, in Part 6, you'll find additional stretches for every part of your body.

You'll notice the following sidebars throughout the book. They highlight certain points to help you get the best results from healthy stretching.

You Heard What?

Some of the misconceptions people have about stretching and what's good for you are truly amazing. In these boxes, I'll deal with those and give the correct information.

Chris's Concerns

Please pay special attention to these boxes. You'll find them whenever I want to tell you something very important about the stretch.

Stretching Strategies

Check these boxes for more information on the healthy stretch you're doing or where to find additional stretches that can help you.

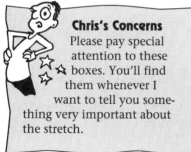

Mr. Stretch Explains

These boxes give easy-to-understand explanations that will help you understand more about healthy stretching.

Acknowledgments

I would like to dedicate this book to my parents, Joseph and Mary Verna, for their encouragement and guidance. I would also like to acknowledge the following individuals: John Smoltz, who took a chance when I first started and who believed in me and helped me grow with new professional clients; his agent, Myles Shoda, who was the first agent to understand and believe in what I was trying to accomplish. To David and Kelly Leadbetter for their hospitality and their belief in me and to Nick Price and Nick Faldo for including me in their careers. To Peter Johnson and IMG for introducing me to Arnold Palmer, Joe Montana, Mike Geminski, and Ivan Lendl. My special thanks to Warren Bosworth who helped me set up my Florida practice and expand the awareness to Ivan Lendl and many other people. To those who helped me become a flexibility specialist— Dr. John Faggert, MD; Dr. Bobby Papton, Ph.D.; Tim Kirschner, A.T.C., Gary Schoenberger, PT; Phil Donley, PT, AT, C. To Howie Bedell for helping me get started as a trainer in professional athletics. To all those who I wouldn't allow to sign my table—Dr. Donald M., Sydney M., Joanne P., David D., Lindsay W., Beth M., and Gina M. Thanks to Mickey and Janice Cartin for the lovely setting and to Arnold Palmer's Bay Hill Club in Orlando, Florida, for all of their help and locations. Special thanks to Bette & Court and Peter Glenn Ski Shops. To Lisa Kopplin for devoting so much time and energy helping me demonstrate the stretches. I also want to thank Dick Staron for having the foresight to get this Guide published and to Kathy Nebenhaus for her incredible executive ability to keep it on track. And one very big special thank you to our editor, Joan Paterson, whose professionalism, friendship, encouragement, and common sense saved the day.

Trademarks

Part 1
Understanding Stretching and Flexibility

Would you like me to start by showing you just how flexible you currently are? If we were together, I could probably tell just by watching you walk into my office. The next best thing, however, is to let me guide you through a simple flexibility self-test. Together we'll be able to pinpoint any problem areas you may have. Don't worry—you're not going to have to change into one of those "open in the back" examination gowns.

Your lifestyle plays a big role in your overall flexibility, along with how you are built and your past physical history. Once we have an understanding of what's causing your flexibility problems, I'll explain how healthy stretching your muscles works and why you should start feeling better once we begin.

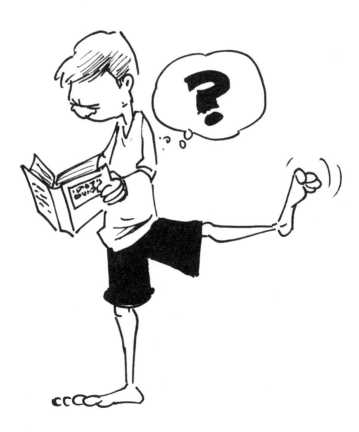

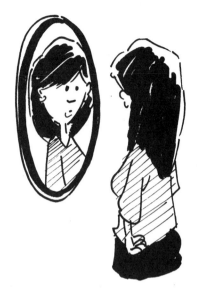

Chapter 1

Here's Looking at You, Kid— Your Flexibility Self-Test

In This Chapter

➤ I'll help you look at yourself like never before

➤ Could your posture be hiding something?

➤ We'll look at how your body is currently moving

➤ Together, we'll determine areas to work on

> You're not supposed to move like the Tin Man in *The Wizard of Oz.*
> —Chris "Mr. Stretch" Verna

You're traveling down the Yellow Brick Road with Dorothy, the Scarecrow, the Cowardly Lion and—the antithesis to flexibility himself—the Tin Man. Even well oiled, he still saunters along stiffly. It's a good thing the Tin Man only asked the Wizard for a heart. Can you imagine the headaches he would have suffered being that tight if he asked for nerves instead?

Using the Tin Man example in my presentations to groups around the country really illustrates how we are not supposed to move. We don't move solidly, instead we rotate or move in circles within our joints (balls and sockets that are part of the bone structure). I'll explain all of this in Chapter 3. But right now, we need to find out about you. How do you move and how flexible are you?

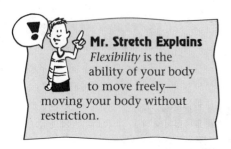

Mr. Stretch Explains
Flexibility is the ability of your body to move freely—moving your body without restriction.

This flexibility test will help identify any problem areas you might have and may turn up a few surprises. Lacking flexibility in a specific area may be coming from some other place than you might think.

If we find that you have limited flexibility in some or even all areas, don't be concerned. You're not a complete physical wreck. I'll suggest some stretches and where to find them in the Guide.

Healthy stretching is easily blended into your daily routine, since you don't need special clothing or equipment. You'll be able to identify yourself in upcoming chapters that deal with lifestyle and sports. The healthy stretches in those chapters will get you back on the road to flexibility. If you still need a little more help, Part 6 features healthy stretches for the exact area you need to work on. Even doing those doesn't take a lot of time, especially as you become more flexible.

I only stretch five minutes a day to maintain my flexibility. But, remember, I know someone in the business. So let's have some fun and get started.

Who's Walking in Your Footsteps?

Let's start by looking at the way you walk. Have you ever wondered who made those strange tracks in the sand or snow when you turn around? You did! In fact those very tracks provide lots of information about some problems with your flexibility. Can you find your tracks in the Photos 1-1 and 1-2?

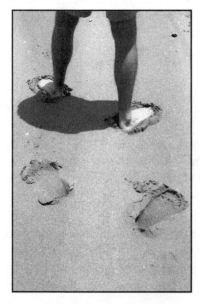

Photo 1-1. Waddling duck.

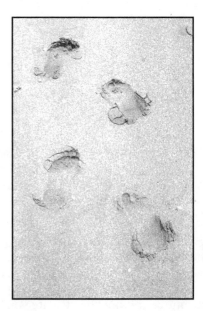

Photo 1-2. Lost pigeon.

Waddling Duck

"I couldn't have made those tracks, a duck must have waddled behind me." If the tracks in Photo 1-1 look familiar and you have a tendency to wear out the outside edges of your heels, it shows you probably have tightness in your hip joint. To confirm this, stand up and look down. Your toes should be somewhat pointed out. If both feet point out the tightness could be in both hip joints. If one foot is fairly straight while the other's pointed out, the pointed-out side usually has the tightness.

The tracks are not caused by just aimlessly wandering down the beach or through the snow. Even if you try to straighten out your feet as you walk, it just won't feel natural and shortly you'll be back to the duck waddle. The tightness is most likely caused by a group of small muscles, the hip rotators, whose job description is to move your foot in and out. These muscles are located under the big muscles of your derrière. I'll bet you thought your ankles were responsible? Wrong!

Stretching Strategies
Okay duck waddler, I have some hip-joint stretches that will get you back on track in Chapter 20. One special exercise that really helps is the Pretzel.

Lost Pigeon

Do your footprints in the sand look like the pigeon tracks in Photo 1-2? Do you normally walk a bit toe in? If you think your ankles are causing you to make these tracks, you're wrong. The real problem usually is a tightness in a group of muscles located in your inner thigh. Trying to walk straighter is not the answer. Healthy stretching the muscle group will improve your flexibility, naturally allowing the foot's return to a more normal position.

Stretching Strategies
Want to get rid of your pigeon tracks? Chapter 20 has some stretches to help you increase the flexibility in your inner thigh.

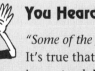

You Heard What?

"Some of the great athletes are somewhat pigeon-toed. How bad can it be?" It's true that certain athletes (usually sprinters) may be somewhat pigeon-toed. Wide receivers in football may also fit into this category. They are superbly conditioned athletes.

Being pigeon-toed, in your case, is not an advantage, but a potential source of injuries. You may not have the strength to avoid the arch, ankle, and knee injuries that can develop.

If Your Posture Could Speak

> ❗ 👦 **Mr. Stretch Explains**
>
> *Your body might be compensating* is an expression I use to help you understand how the body adjusts itself to compensate for losses in flexibility. If you notice one shoulder is lower than the other, the body may be compensating for a neck area problem, not a shoulder problem. The same is true about certain pains. Where it's hurting might not be the source of why it's hurting.

Your posture, the way you stand and sit, can also tell us quite a lot. You'll need a full-length mirror so you can evaluate your posture. Compare it with Photos 1-3 and 1-4 as I guide you along.

I've placed a line down the center of our model, Lisa, as a reference point. Don't tape your mirror at home to simulate this but I do suggest hanging a piece of rope over or in front of the mirror. Weight it at the bottom by tying on something heavy so it hangs straight down, or just visualize the line.

You've probably never used a mirror to look at yourself the way I want you to now. Normally the mirror is used for specific purposes, like shaving, makeup, doing your hair, and dressing. Now I want you to *really* look at yourself, as if I were with you, so we can both analyze what you see. Remember, it's not always what you see that's causing a loss of flexibility. *Your body might be compensating* by adjusting its position.

The Statue of Liberty

Look at Photo 1-3 and stand the same way in front of a mirror. Begin by trying to line yourself up so the rope, or imaginary vertical line, starts at the top of your head, hangs down though the center of your eyes, the center of your chin, and follows down through the center of your body. This straight line is a reference point to determine if your body is *symmetrical*, or balanced evenly on both sides of the line. Classic architecture is symmetrical. You've had your body for a while so it's like classic architecture, or should be.

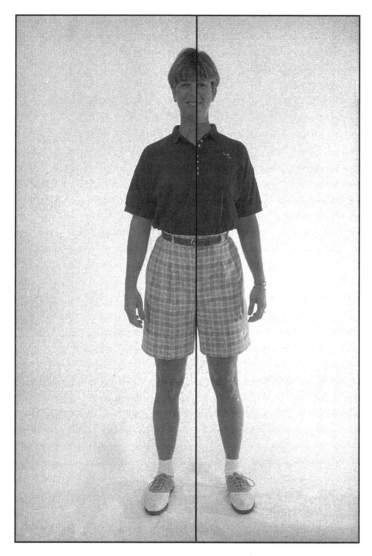

Photo 1-3. Good posture: As you look in the mirror, concentrate on the top of the shoulders and the outside part of your hips. Are they both level?

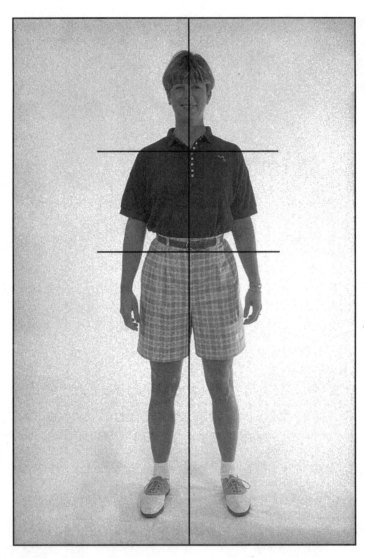

Photo 1-4. Visualize imaginary horizontal lines across your shoulders and your hips. Ideally, each horizontal imaginary line should form a "T" with the hanging vertical line.

Leaning Tower of Pisa

If your imaginary shoulder line is not forming a "T" with the vertical line as in Photo 1-4, you may be really tight on the opposite side of your neck. For instance, if you're leaning to the right, the tightness generally is on the left side of your neck. So it's not that your right shoulder is low, the tightness may be causing your left shoulder to be high. If you're leaning to the left, the opposite may be the case. Usually it's an upper body tightness if the hips are even and the shoulders are tilted. However, if you sit down and the shoulders become even, the tightness should be in your hips.

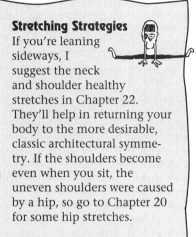

Stretching Strategies
If you're leaning sideways, I suggest the neck and shoulder healthy stretches in Chapter 22. They'll help in returning your body to the more desirable, classic architectural symmetry. If the shoulders become even when you sit, the uneven shoulders were caused by a hip, so go to Chapter 20 for some hip stretches.

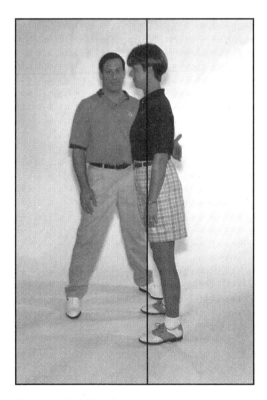

Photo 1-5. Tilted posture.

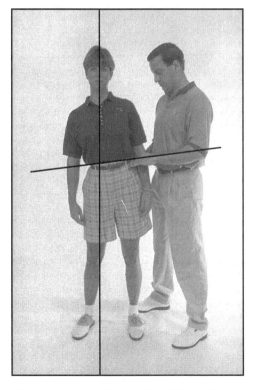

Photo 1-6. One hip higher. Notice how Lisa is leaning to her right.

You have one hip higher than the other (Photo 1-6) if you can't form a "T" with the imaginary and hanging lines. Let's assume your right hip is higher. The cause is usually lower-right side back tightness. The muscle has tightened and become shorter. It can also be caused by a tilting of the pelvis (the bone structure that forms the hips). The hip flexor muscle group may be the culprit.

Stretching Strategies
Hips tilting? Chapter 20 and Chapter 21 both have healthy stretches that will pinpoint the muscle groups you need to stretch.

How Do You Look From the Side?

Now turn yourself sideways like Lisa in Photo 1-7, so the hanging rope lines up with your ears, shoulders and point of your hips. The question is does it line up like Photo 1-7 or are you hunched forward as in Photo 1-8?

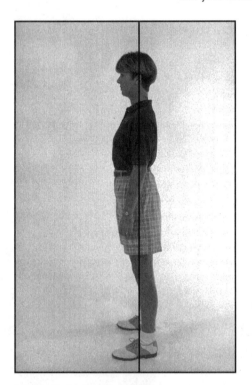

Photo 1-7. Good posture.

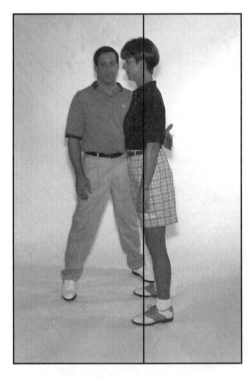

Photo 1-8. Forward tilted posture.

You may not even be aware you're hunched forward. Your body may have compensated with this position for so long it's become a normal feeling. Are you aware of some sensitivity if you're touched on the front of your chest where it meets your arm?

Knees and Ankles, the Propellers

It's not unusual to have some sort of knee and ankle problems. After all, they form the support for your body's weight and are responsible for literally propelling you along life's path. Also life's fairway, life's tennis court, and…enough, I think you've got the picture.

In some cases, injuries are caused by problems in other areas. Your body, compensating for problems in knees or ankles, can cause other problems to develop in the upper body. Some compensation! If the brain had to support the weight, maybe it would review its decisions.

Getting a Knee Up

You can leave the mirror and head over to a doorway as we check your knee flexibility. Let's test your left side first.

Stretching Strategies
Chest and shoulder healthy stretches will lead you back to Statue of Liberty straightness. You can find them in Chapters 21 and 22.

Chris's Concerns
When doing the Knee-Up test, please don't reach back with your body to grab your foot. Stop this test immediately if that's the only way you can reach it. You already know you are much too tight. If you lay on your side and reach for your ankle, you can do this test lying down. I suggest, however, you proceed to the Knee Differential test and locate the cause of the tightness.

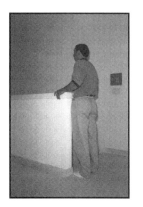 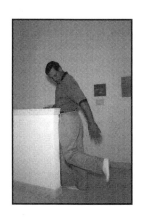 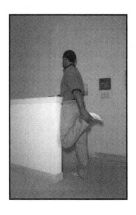

Photo 1-9 (Left). Place the front of your left hip and left knee up against a wall or door molding. Photo 1-10 (Middle). Reach down with your left hand as you pick up your left foot, grasping it in front of your ankle. Photo 1-11 (Right). If you can touch your left heel to your derrière, that's good flexibility.

Repeat the test with the right knee by placing the front of the right hip and knee against the molding.

If you feel a pull in the top of the knee to the front of your thigh as you are trying to bring the foot toward your derrière, stop. You have discovered limited flexibility. Remember how far you were able to bring it back this time. Now we have to determine if the limited flexibility is related to the knee or a group of muscles that connect with the hip. Do the differential test next. Then repeat this test with the right knee by placing the front of the right hip and knee against the molding.

Knee Differential Test

Let's find the cause of your limited knee flexibility. If you had to stop somewhere along the way in the previous exercise, it's time to find what's causing it, the knee or the hip.

How far you're able to move your left foot determines how good the flexibility of the hip muscle group is. If you can't move your knee six to 10 inches away from the wall, the tightness would seem more related to your hip.

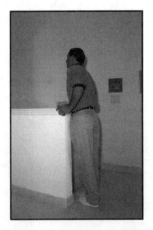

Photo 1-12. Stand in the same position you started with in Photo 1-9.

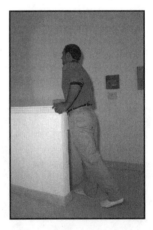

Photo 1-13. Move your left foot back and away from the wall.

Ankles Away

You can use the lower step of a staircase, a step on your porch, or even place several wide, thick books on the floor to test the flexibility of your ankles.

The angle the lowered ankle forms tells us about your flexibility. A 45-degree angle is very good. If you can't get your heel to go past the step, don't force it because you have very limited flexibility. Now repeat this test for your other ankle.

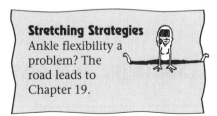

Chris's Concerns
Never push the ankle down when you do this test. Relax it down as far as it wants to go. People injure themselves by forcing the body into positions it can't reach naturally.

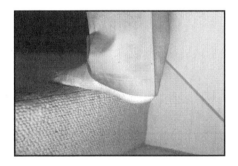

Photo 1-14. Start by standing backward on a bottom step. Put the weight on the ball of your foot.

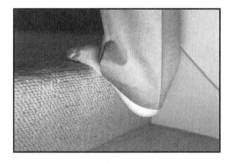

Photo 1-15. Let your ankle go down, but don't push it down.

Okay, You're Not Elvis, But How Flexible Are Your Hips?

In the interest of our working together I'm not going to make any hip jokes here. So instead I'll be more clinical and tell you the hips are located at the center of body movement. If you're athletic you already have a pretty good idea of how the hips should move in your favorite sport. In our day-to-day lives they are extremely important and tightness in the hip muscle groups usually causes compensation problems elsewhere. I've previously explained how ankle and knee problems can directly be related to hip problems too.

Stretching Strategies
Ankle flexibility a problem? The road leads to Chapter 19.

For this test, you need a straight-back chair, and this time you get to sit down.

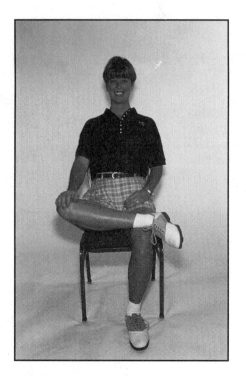

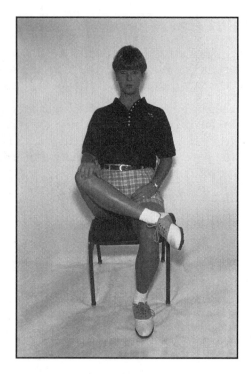

Photo 1-16. Sit in the chair with your derrière and shoulders touching the back of the chair. Rest your right ankle on your left thigh so the knee forms a 90-degree angle.

Photo 1-17. See the height the right knee is above the left, indicating limited flexibility in the right hip.

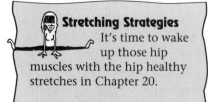

Stretching Strategies
It's time to wake up those hip muscles with the hip healthy stretches in Chapter 20.

The height your right knee is above your left knee determines your flexibility. Photo 1-16 is an example of good flexibility. Now test your other hip by reversing legs.

With limited flexibility in the right hip as shown in Photo 1-17, you'll probably also feel a pulling sensation in your right hip joint or in your derrière.

Shoulders—You've Been Carrying the World on Them

Think of the shoulders and neck and you think tension, tension, tension. Tightness is not unusual in the shoulders, but let's test them for flexibility, starting with Shoulder Test #1.

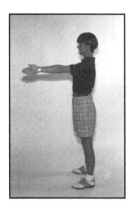
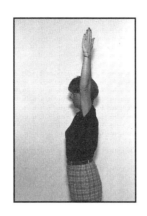
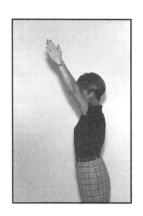

Photo 1-18 (Left). Test one arm at a time by extending your left arm out straight and parallel to the floor. Photo 1-19 (Middle). Keeping your arm straight, raise it as far as you can above your head. This photo shows an example of outstanding shoulder flexibility. Photo 1-20 (Right). This photo shows an example of limited shoulder flexibility.

If you were raising your arm and felt increased tightness in the top of your shoulder, your shoulder flexibility may be limited. If you also feel it in your neck, you probably have a neck flexibility problem. In any case, take note of how far you were able to raise each arm.

We've tested the shoulder for up and down flexibility. Now let's see how you do with each shoulder rotating side to side. Try Shoulder Test #2.

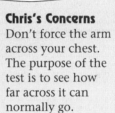

Chris's Concerns
Don't force the arm across your chest. The purpose of the test is to see how far across it can normally go.

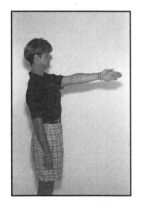
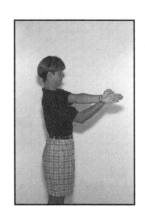
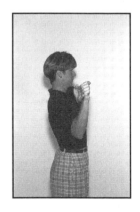

Photo 1-21 (Left). Extend your arm out straight so it forms a 90-degree angle to your body and is parallel to the floor. Photo 1-22 (Middle). Place the back of the wrist of your other hand on the far side of the extended arm on your wrist. Photo 1-23 (Right). Keeping the extended arm straight, gently push the arm across your chest with your other arm. This photo shows good flexibility.

15

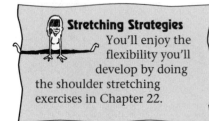

Stretching Strategies
You'll enjoy the flexibility you'll develop by doing the shoulder stretching exercises in Chapter 22.

Stretching Strategies
If you can't extend your elbows out straight, I suggest you do the elbow exercises in Chapter 23 and the shoulder stretches in Chapter 22. Elbow and shoulder flexibility problems are very often linked.

Photo 1-24. Good elbow flexibility.

If you have excellent flexibility, you should be able to have the extended arm touch the opposite shoulder.

Elbows and Wrists

You're getting a better understanding of your overall flexibility as we move from area to area. Even great athletes have flexibility problems, so don't think you're a total wreck. The great thing about healthy stretching is you won't have to devote a lot of time to doing the exercises. Healthy stretching blends into your life.

Are You an Elbow Bender?

The elbow test is quite simple but you should do this in front of the mirror. Extend both arms in front of you and toward the mirror with your palms up just like in Photo 1-24.

The flexibility is fine if you can fully extend your arms, but limited if you can't. Don't force them to get straight, just extend them normally.

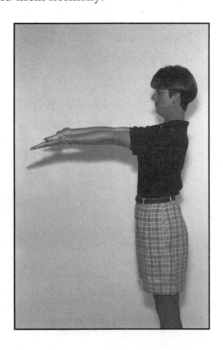

Do Your Wrists Have Trouble Waving Goodbye?

We take wrist flexibility for granted. Yet it's not unusual for the wrists to be somewhat restricted by a variety of things. Past injuries when we were younger, or even problems resulting from repeated tasks can be the cause. We'll deal with some of those problems in Chapter 8, but for now, let's check your wrist flexibility.

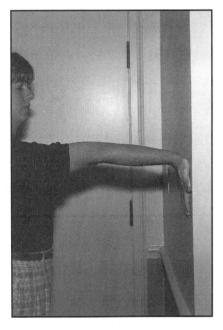

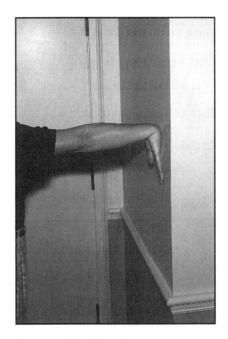

Photo 1-25. To test for wrist flexibility, stand within arm's length of a wall. Extend your arm out so that your palm is touching the wall.

Photo 1-26. This time when you extend your arm out try to place the back of your hand on the wall.

If you can get the heel of your palm to touch the wall, your flexibility is fine. If not, it's limited. Don't forget to test the other wrist. Now test both wrists again, but this time for flexibility in the other direction. If you can do it, your flexibility is fine. If not, you have a wrist flexibility problem.

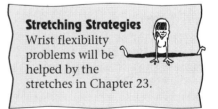

Stretching Strategies
Wrist flexibility problems will be helped by the stretches in Chapter 23.

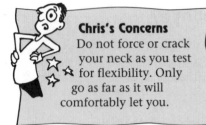

Sticking Your Neck Out

If you're a pain in the neck there's nothing I can do for you. But if you have one, I can help. Neck pain is almost always caused by neck flexibility problems with the shoulder sometimes playing a role. We need the mirror again to test. Start with Neck Test #1.

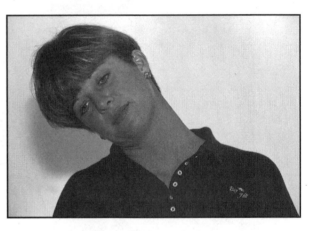

Photo 1-28. Without moving your shoulders, try to gently touch your ear to your shoulder. This photo shows good neck flexibility in this direction.

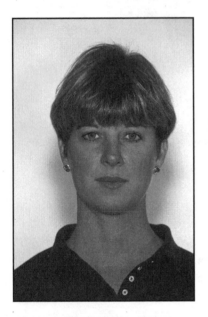

Photo 1-27. Start by facing your mirror.

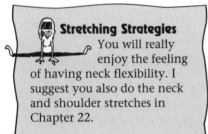

Be sure to test the opposite side. It's a likely indication you have neck flexibility problems if you can't get your ear about halfway to your shoulder. You'll feel the tightness on the opposite side of the neck. Remember how far you went for future reference. Now try Neck Test #2.

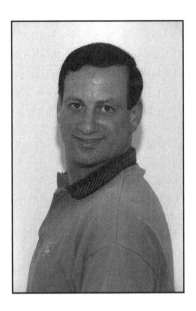

Photo 1-29. With your shoulder 90 degrees to a mirror, gently turn your head toward the mirror as far as possible or until you can get your chin over your shoulder. This photo shows excellent neck flexibility in this direction. Be sure to do this stretch in both directions.

The Physical Part of the Test Is Over

Flexibility is something that can be easily lost, as you may have noticed from this physical part of the test. We have an indication as to where your flexibility problems are, but I need some more information as to what may have caused them. Chapter 2 will help us learn a little more about your past physical problems, body type, and symptoms of pains you may be feeling. It's important to understand why and where you have reduced flexibility.

Healthy stretching can soon have you feeling better. You don't have to be an athlete to discover the benefits of healthy stretching. All of us move every day; we can do it stiffly and develop problems or we can rotate flexibly through life.

The Least You Need to Know

➤ Flexibility is the ability of your body to move freely.

➤ The body is not designed to move in a straight line. We rotate and move in circles within our joints.

➤ You may think you know the cause of a problem, but it may be the result of something else. The body makes compensations to get you through daily life.

➤ After taking the rotational flexibility test you now have a clear understanding of just how flexible you are.

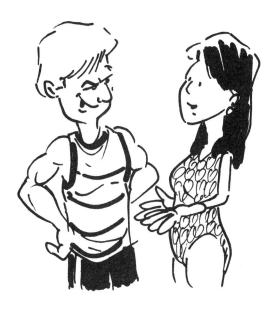

Chapter 2

Tell Me a Little About Yourself!

In This Chapter

➤ Your history may have left a trail to your flexibility problems

➤ Lifestyle affects your flexibility

➤ How past injuries may have caused a loss of flexibility

➤ Why certain pains may be sending out an SOS for stretching

In Chapter 1 you were able to physically determine your own flexibility and began to develop an understanding as to some problem areas. Now, it's time to put on our houndstooth double-brimmed hats and play Sherlock Holmes as we delve into your personal lifestyle and history searching for clues to the cause. Yes, my clever friend, you left a trail behind you and I'm not going to rest until I track down and expose to the cruel light of day the reasons for your flexibility problems. It's elementary, my dear reader, purely deductive reasoning.

Seriously, our lifestyle, history, and body type actually do have a big influence on our flexibility. Have you heard the expression "use it or lose it"? In the case of flexibility, it's very true because our *muscles* have a tendency to forget how to work, if we don't use

Mr. Stretch Explains
Muscles vary in shape and size and are made up of strands of tissue. Large muscles like the hamstrings located in the back of your upper leg create motion while other muscles have responsibilities you can't control.

them, forcing body compensation to help us move. I'll help you understand more about this in Chapter 3.

Once you couple the understanding of where your loss of flexibility is (Chapter 1) with how your lifestyle and history contribute to it, I'll really be able to help you on the road back toward regaining it.

Are You a Sitter?

A simple way to start is to determine whether you sit most of the day or spend it on your feet. Sitting may be work related or by choice. Does this definition list of a *sitter* describe you?

➤ You sit at a desk most of the day typing or on the phone.

➤ You think you're constantly on the go but spend most of your day in meetings.

➤ You have a hectic schedule but you spend over half a day on a plane traveling, several times per week.

➤ Your work requires long hours each day in a car or truck.

➤ Regardless of your occupation and leisure time you honestly know you tend to sit for over half the day.

A sitter's muscles are shortened for long periods of time. Our bodies adapt to our lifestyle and sitting says to the muscles "shorten to the length I need to sit." So if you sit for a long time your muscles become used to that shorter length. Just because your mind's working doesn't mean your muscles are.

Let's say you work in an office five days a week and then, on the weekend, you like to do some gardening that requires bending or recreational activities that include running,

Stretching Strategies
In Part 3, we'll be much more specific about how your life and work styles have affected your flexibility. We'll also demonstrate some healthy stretches that take only a few minutes and can be done any place you're sitting.

walking, or swinging movements. Those, used to sitting length, muscles are not going to make the necessary changes to accommodate the one or two days of the weekend since they have developed other habits five days a week.

Now you know what's causing your aching back or the strained muscle in the back of your leg. The strain's caused by a slight tearing of the muscle fiber as you forced it to quickly lengthen beyond what it's normally used to. You can't change the need for sitting most of the time but you can incorporate some stretching exercises that will help your muscles know all week long they also need to be able to adapt to your weekend lifestyle.

Are You a Stander?

If you're on your feet for more than an hour at a time and for extended periods of the day, you fit into the standers category. Teachers, construction workers, retail sales people, and health care providers will probably fit into this group. Your body has adapted your muscles to the standing and walking positions and since certain muscles have to support the body's weight for long periods of time, this *fatigues the muscles* used for these purposes. You've heard the expression "sit down and take a load off"?

As a stander you probably have some lower back discomfort and stiff knees from time to time, usually a result of muscle fatigue. If you also carry heavy objects, the added weight is supported by muscles already under the burden of carrying you around all day. They let you know, from time to time, "Hey, I need some help here." You can send some help by stretching the muscles and re-educating them to return to their normal length.

Mr. Stretch Explains
Fatigues the muscles means the muscle weakens to the point where it can't fully support the load that's being put on it. When a muscle *fatigues*, it actually shortens. Healthy stretching re-educates muscles, returning them to proper length.

Have You Ever Been Injured?

Flexibility can also be affected and influenced by your past history of injury. If you've suffered a severe injury that required extensive medical care and rehabilitation, you're already well aware of what loss of flexibility can mean and how hard you had to work to regain it.

If you ever incurred a *fracture,* a broken bone that required a cast, or suffered a muscle or *ligament* strain in the past, you may not be aware it may still be causing a flexibility problem for you. In fact, the problem may be in an area unrelated to your original injury.

Mr. Stretch Explains
Ligaments are tough bands of tissue that connect bones together or sup-port an organ in place. Bones are connected to each other at a point called a *joint.* Hips, knees, and elbows are all examples of *joints.*

Bone Fractures

Fractured bones usually require a cast to be worn for a period of time. Consequently, a few flexibility problems arise. Muscle groups that work with the bone to move it *atrophy*, which means they get smaller and shrink because they are not being used. Your muscles, along with the involved ligaments and tendons, all protect the bone as part of the body's natural defense. Unfortunately, if the cast is on for an extended period of time, the joint that has been immobilized or restricted from movement stiffens severely, restricting flexibility.

Rehabilitation usually consists of stretching exercises that re-educate the affected muscle groups, letting them know it's okay to get back to work and allow the joint to move more freely, regaining its intended flexibility.

Muscle Strains

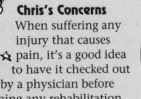

Chris's Concerns
When suffering any injury that causes pain, it's a good idea to have it checked out by a physician before beginning any rehabilitation on your own. While you may think it's only a slight muscle tear, the pain may be coming from fractures or other problems that physicians are trained to diagnose.

Your body does not want to cause further damage to itself after an injury. If you strain a muscle, creating a slight tear, the muscle will go into an immediate shortened state, referred to as a *muscle spasm,* to protect itself from further tearing and injury.

The muscle will hold or stay in that shortened state until you help it learn, by stretching, to re-establish its length, allowing proper function to return. It's imperative that you immediately start trying to rehabilitate the muscle right away because the *scar tissue* (the new tissue that knits the torn muscle fibers back together) that forms as a result of the healing process may prevent you from having that muscle return to its proper length ever again. Stretching exercises should be part of the rehabilitation process.

Ligament Strains

You already know ligaments attach bones to bones. Unfortunately, once a ligament is sprained it permanently changes shape, never returning to its normal structure. Let's say, for example, you turned your ankle spraining a ligament. Since that ligament can't ever be the same, you'll have a tendency to keep spraining the same ankle, since it may be weakened.

Mr. Stretch Explains
Tendons hold the muscles to the bone. Made up of fibrous connective tissue or tough cords, tendons also transmit the forces muscles exert.

The body, compensating for the sprained ligament, asks the muscles to assist the ligaments. Attached to the bones by *tendons,* muscles need to be educated with healthy stretching, once given this extra duty. When the ankle starts getting itself into trouble, educated muscles will help keep the ankle in alignment. If your muscles are not stretched and strong, they won't be able to help the damaged ligament hold and another ankle injury will probably occur.

Be Honest Now...How Are You Built?

Your body size characteristics and makeup have a lot to do with your flexibility too. For example, you could be a weight lifter with an incredible physique but, if you built yourself up without also stretching the muscles, you're probably very inflexible.

Pick out the category you most closely match. If you have trouble identifying with any in this group, you might find yourself described in the lifestyle choices category we'll cover next. Both your physical stature and, to some extent, your lifestyle play a role in how flexible you currently are.

You Heard What?

It's a common misconception that overweight people are inflexible and thin people are always flexible. I've discovered that some of the finest athletes in the world have suffered with inflexibility because they never stretched and trained their muscles properly. Being overweight for them is not a problem. Flexibility is created and maintained by properly keeping your muscles activated by stretching them regardless of your weight.

NFL Lineman

If you're tall with a big waist, broad shoulders, thick ankles, wrists, and big legs, this is your body type category. Your body mass requires a lot more work from the muscles to overcome your body weight. Muscles enable the body to move by contracting, producing *tension,* the force generating the bones to move. Big guys require a lot more tension to create the momentum and speed needed to move.

You may think you're inflexible, big guy, because it's difficult to get into the positions to stretch—but it's not your weight causing it. One of my most flexible clients is former NFL lineman John Offerdahl of the Miami Dolphins.

Marathon Runner

You may not actually run in marathons but if you have thin wrists, and ankles, are thinly muscled with slender hips and long bones this is your body type. You're probably very active but that doesn't mean you're the ultimate example of flexibility. Some of the tightest athletes I've worked with are actually in this category.

It may stem from the fact that marathon runners take their slimness along with athletic ability to mean they must be flexible. I've found including healthy stretching routines enable people in this category to improve their performance by allowing their talents to come through with the added benefit of reducing injury potential.

Workout Woman

This is your category if you are a woman who does some form of exercise four or five times a week. It could be aerobics or strength training.

All of these exercises require an active use of the muscles and just doing the warm-up exercises is not enough to properly stretch the muscles. I know you

Chris's Concerns
After strenuous exercise your muscles become fatigued and shorten. Stretching re-educates them into resuming their proper length, helping to reduce day-after stiffness experienced by so many people.

also do cool-down exercises, but one of the big things I'm going to cover in Chapter 4 is the need to stretch the muscles before and after to prevent stiffness.

Supermodel

A supermodel type is a woman who has always been naturally thin and doesn't usually have to work hard to keep her figure in shape. There is the tendency to take the body for granted, believing it will always stay that way, especially when they're younger.

As the supermodel body types get older, they fail to understand why they can't get their bodies back into that shape. Could the reason be when you're given something and didn't have to work for it, it's very difficult to keep it? It seems, on the other hand, that supermodel body types who have worked hard to keep fit have stayed in shape for longer periods of time.

Do I Really Have to Tell You, Mr. Stretch?

Both men and women comprise this category. It's not that you don't care about your body but taking the time to stay in shape doesn't appeal to you. I could tell you about all the bad side effects and potential illnesses that can affect individuals who don't want to stay in shape, but I won't.

You're not alone, there are more people who don't want to exercise than those who do. They think it's time-consuming, unpleasant, and only for athletes. Remember, since you now have this Guide, I've become your personal flexibility trainer. I assure you that stretching will take hardly any time and you'll feel better almost immediately.

You won't have to purchase any expensive endorsed gym equipment or clothing: You're all set now. This is not the touch your toes or jumping jacks exercises people associate with stretching. Instead it's exercises that trigger energy and you'll be surprised how good you can feel right from the start.

Tell Me How You Play!

Your leisure time is another source providing clues to how your body is used and how muscles have to adapt. We all want the most from life and with hectic schedules our leisure time has to be crammed in. You may be a person who likes to do something every day, like run or walk, or you may have to limit your activities to the weekends. Let's find the lifestyle and exercise category you come closest to.

Endurance Sports

You're an endurance sports person if you:

➤ Take long walks at least five times a week.

➤ Follow a regular program of running or cycling.

➤ Fit into the Workout Woman or Marathon Runner category.

➤ Adhere to a workout program a minimum of five days a week.

Many distance runners generally don't stretch, preferring to warm up and stretch out while they're running. They can get away with that in high school but as they get into their 30s and 40s it gets tougher to keep going and prevent muscle damage. When the same muscle groups are repeatedly utilized, other muscle groups need some attention. Many champions in endurance sports keep achieving higher and higher performance levels because they include stretching as a part of their training.

Chris's Concerns
People who partici-
pate in endurance
sports tend to focus
more on the activity
they're doing, when
they also need to make sure
their muscles can keep
fulfilling the demands asked
of them.

In a sport like running, the most important piece of equipment is the body. Yes, I've seen the ads about footwear too, but something has to propel the feet: That's the muscles' job. So doesn't it make sense to keep them tuned and stretched to obtain maximum performance? If you're in this category, it's imperative to let me help you with some stretches that will keep you active for years.

Aerobic Sports

If quick action sports that include running are the way you like to spend your leisure time, this is your category. These sports get your heart rate up and feature quick bursts of energy along with some sustained movement. Tennis, basketball, and some walking are examples, as are stationary bikes, climbing machines, and, of course, aerobics classes. The key is you have to participate several times a week, not just occasionally.

The very nature of the activities pursued by this group requires the use of many different muscle groups for short periods of time, creating potential for a wide range of muscle and joint stiffness. If this is your category, you may be fitness aware—but stretching before and after your exercise may improve your performance and help protect you from injury.

You Heard What?
It's a common misconception to think that just because you exercised for only a short period of time you didn't fatigue the muscles. It's also not true to think the more you use muscles, the more flexible you are. Muscles get fatigued and shorten with exercise, regardless of the duration depending on your fitness level. If you don't keep the muscles stretched, they'll develop new patterns to stay short, restricting your flexibility.

Weekend Warrior

This category probably applies to most people. Is this you?

➤ You play tennis once or twice a week.

➤ You participate in a regular weekly softball or basketball game.

➤ Weekends are great for water skiing, or rollerblading around the park a few times.

➤ You do something athletic once or twice a week at full speed.

You can't disguise being a Weekend Warrior. You're the one limping and moaning, taking some type of pain medication, and smelling like wintergreen from the rub-on deep-heating muscle creams. I understand you have limited time so you have to get right at it.

Pharmaceutical companies love you, and so does the medical profession because the number of weekend warrior injuries is staggering. What do you expect if you're sedentary most of the week but, when the weekend arrives, you become a raving sports maniac?

Chris's Concerns
Before beginning any intense exercise, find the healthy stretches in the chapter dealing with the sport. Do the stretches before and especially after the exercise to educate the muscle to return to its proper length, preventing injury, soreness, and a loss of flexibility.

Here's what causes the problems. Because your normal lifestyle educated your muscles to function in a certain manner, getting revved up and exercising furiously confuses them, creating indecision on how to adapt quickly. Confusion in the muscles results in a loss of flexibility while increasing potential for injuries.

Making matters worse, Weekend Warriors try to do one or two warm-up exercises, like bending way over bouncing their bodies to touch their toes, mistakenly believing they're stretching them. That, my friends, is not healthy stretching. This Guide will be extremely beneficial if you do some healthy stretches for a short time every day. You'll be in shape for the weekend in a brand new category: Mr. Stretch's new and improved Weekend Warrior.

I Get a Round In!

You occasionally go out and do something. It may be playing golf or taking a walk once or twice a month. Your regular exercise may include walking from building to building or down the street for lunch. You may not have realized, until taking the flexibility test in Chapter 1, just how inflexible you are.

If this is your category, you need to educate your muscles with some healthy stretching. I know you don't value the benefits of exercise—but you enjoy feeling good, don't you? Stretching is different from heavy exercise. You can even do a stretch or two when you're in your car or waiting for a cab. Stretching won't infringe on your lifestyle, but it will make you feel so good you may want to take the next step and become my version of the new and improved Weekend Warrior.

Well, Mr. Stretch, I Have This Great Couch!

You don't have to be curled up on your couch watching television to be a couch potato. If you find yourself spending loads of time at your computer or spending your time doing something that doesn't let you move, this is your category.

This category also includes some senior citizens who mostly stay inside sitting or others who always feel so tired they don't have the energy to exercise. The problem is you're in a cycle: The more you sit, the worse your body feels and the less you want to do.

The first stretching exercise I have for you can't wait for the later chapters. It's not difficult either. Just start immediately moving your body. Don't keep the potato chips next to you, get up and take small portions from the kitchen, making several trips. In other words, try to make things a little less convenient so you have to expend some energy and make your muscles move.

I could tell you where in the Guide you'll find some stretches to do while sitting on the couch, but I'd rather you work on finger and wrist flexibility by stretching your fingers as you turn the pages searching.

I'm Not Your Mom, But Where Does it Hurt?

SOS. SOS. SOS. "Can anybody hear me? This is your body. Hey, I need some help here. I'll teach you not to ignore me. How about a little neck ache. Aha, that got some attention. Now, a nice throbbing shoulder should get some response."

There's not some self-centered evil gremlin controlling your body, but pain is a way for the body to let you know you have a problem. It's not unusual to have some occasional aches and pains. I trust you already understand that severe or worsening pain requires seeing a physician.

If, on the other hand, your discomfort is something involving muscles and joints, healthy stretching can help silence the SOS signal your body occasionally sends out, interrupting a good night's sleep.

I Have This Pain in My Neck

The first thing you need to tell me is what position you sleep in at night: on your back, side, or on your stomach. If you sleep on your stomach, you're twisting your neck in the wrong positions all night long. If you sleep on your back, it's not as bad but you're flattening your spine. Sleeping on your side provides the ideal position: It keeps the stress off the spine. Sometimes putting a pillow on the side, by your stomach, helps keep you from rolling over. The type of pillow you use for your head must be able to support your neck and be comfortable.

Chris's Concerns
If the pain starts in your neck and goes down your arm, it's something more serious and you need to see a physician. If it's in your neck and upper back, try stretching in the morning after a warm shower.

Can I Exchange This Back for One That Works?

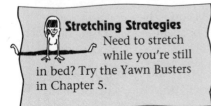

Stretching Strategies
Need to stretch while you're still in bed? Try the Yawn Busters in Chapter 5.

If you've suffered from chronic backache but your physician can't find anything wrong, the discomfort is most likely coming from your muscles and/or it's stress-related. Stretching can really help. Are you stiff in the morning when you try to get out of bed? You need to stretch before you even put your feet on the floor.

I Love Standing for Five Hours on Cross-Country Flights!

This is my cute way of saying that sitting for hours is uncomfortable. If you've been checked out by your doctor and know nothing is seriously wrong with you, the problem is a loss of flexibility in your hip joints caused by the muscles on one side being tighter than the other side. Both sides could be tight but it's worse to have one side tight than to have both sides tight. The stiffness usually comes from the muscles in front; that's why you feel better when you stand up because you're stretching the muscles.

Part of the problem may be the way you sit. Your sitting position in the car, for example, may be aggravating the muscles. The leg may be slightly turned while you're sitting and you're pushing the accelerator and brake with one foot. How you sit when reading or watching television is also important. Do you have something in your pocket that's pinching, like a wallet, causing discomfort as the muscles react? Healthy stretching should really help you.

Is That Your Knees or Pipes Creaking?

Knee problems are usually a result of poor hip flexibility, in particular the outer and inner thigh. Those muscles groups are attached to your hip and to your knee. If the muscles are tight, the knee is restricted to a forward and backward motion without any balance side to side, putting it under pressure.

It's like walking on stilts and people who aren't good on stilts fall over. The body compensates to provide balance, unfortunately creating problems for other muscle groups. Healthy stretching can re-educate all the various muscles groups returning flexibility to your knee.

I'd Like to Sue This Ankle for Non-Support!

In the injury section of this chapter, you learned that if you sprain your ankle and damage a ligament, the ligament never returns to its original shape. Body compensation requires muscles to take on some extra duty to prevent the ankle from turning over.

If you have a tendency to trip, turn your ankle, or stumble when the terrain changes even a little bit, now you know why. Healthy stretching keeps muscles in good shape to give you the support you need.

How Do the French Say "Everywhere"?

If it seems like you have aches and pains everywhere, you really need to have a professional person help get you started. A flexibility specialist can help take the pressure off your bones by helping you stretch the various muscle groups. Some may be listed as sports rehabilitation therapists. My suggestion is to really talk to your doctor and explain exactly how you feel and ask for some recommendations.

The Least You Need to Know

➤ Your past history and lifestyle affect your flexibility.

➤ Muscles fatigue and shorten when used and need to be re-educated by healthy stretching to return to their proper function.

➤ Muscles adapt to the length that's usually required by your lifestyle. That's why you can injure yourself when you play or attempt other forms of movement.

➤ Healthy stretching keeps the various muscle groups ready for when you need them.

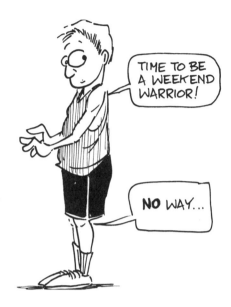

Chapter 3

Your Body's Political System: How it Should Work Together

In This Chapter

➤ A political system of flexibility

➤ Bones, muscles, and joints propelling you along life's highway

➤ Some of your muscles may be on vacation

➤ How healthy stretching re-educates your muscles

Now that you've taken your flexibility test and discovered how history, lifestyle, and injuries play a role in the total picture, how about some in-depth, highly technical information loaded with 26-letter words about how the body works. I saw that yawn and furrowed brow!

Seriously though, it does help if you have some very basic understanding of how muscles, bones, and joints are supposed to interact, creating the 100-percent-flexible individual. Actually, that condition would be worse than being stiff since we still need to stand, move, and support ourselves. With total flexibility, we would be collapsing all over the place. So there is a happy medium.

Maybe the best way to understand the various roles muscles, bones, and joints play is to compare flexibility with another "perfect" working system, our government. Let's call bones the Executive Branch, muscles the Legislative Branch, and joints the Judiciary. And, just as for our government, we need to have something that ideally defines the roles of each.

The Constitution of Flexibility

We, the users of our bodies, in order to create a perfect union of ideal flexibility allowing us to pursue life, liberty, and recreational endeavors, hereby decree the following:

➤ That muscles and bones shall form the musculoskeletal system of our bodies.

➤ The responsibility of the bones shall be to provide support and posture for the body.

➤ The responsibility of the muscles shall be to provide the body with the ability to move.

➤ That, where two bones come together, it shall be called a joint and that connecting the bones shall be the responsibilities of the ligaments with the muscles also providing connection assistance.

➤ The joint shall provide the final decision as to whether the muscles are allowing the bones to properly rotate, ensuring perfect flexibility.

Ideally, that's how the three should work together. As we've learned, both with government and our bodies, that's not always the case. Sometimes history and external influences corrupt the system. Just as we're vigilant and watch our government closely, making changes with elections, we can also make changes if our flexibility is not the best we should expect. Should the problem be muscle-related, the changes can be made with healthy stretching.

Bones: The Executive Branch

Just like the Executive Branch of government (where you find the President and the structure of the various agencies) the bones make up the body's foundation with more than 200 bones making up the human skeleton. While providing support for the body's weight, they also provide protection for the body's internal organs. As an example, bones making up the skull protect the brain while bones making up the rib cage protect the lungs and heart.

Bones are connected to each other by very inelastic connective tissue called ligaments. And while not all bones are designed to move, like the bones making up the protective part of the skull, some must move if you intend to walk and play. The femur, sometimes called the thighbone, is an example of bone that must move. It's connected to your pelvis, the big wide bone structure also called your hips, and to the tibia, the bone often called the shinbone. Figure 3-1 shows the ilium bone of the pelvis and the femur connected at the hip joint by ligaments.

The femur is shaped differently at both ends. Where it meets your pelvis it's shaped more like a ball to fit into the socket of the pelvis. Where the two bones come together is called the hip joint. However the end, where it meets the tibia, looks more like a socket. The joint where the femur and the tibia come together is the knee.

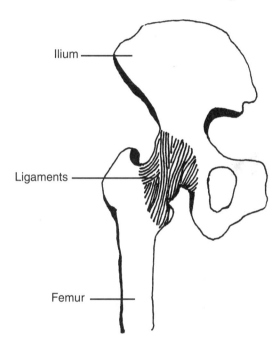

Ilium

Ligaments

Femur

Figure 3-1. Hip joint ligaments.

Muscles: The Legislative Branch

Using our government analogy example, muscles comprise the Legislative Branch (where you find Congress) and the similarities between the two are fascinating. Muscles sometimes work and sometimes go on vacation at the expense of our flexibility. Sometimes they work together and sometimes they're in a state of confusion. Muscles are supposed to be responsive to our needs but, as in government, that can sometimes be a problem.

You Heard What?

If you think all muscles are the same, you're wrong. While we have three muscle groups, we only have the ability to control one of them, the *skeletal muscles*. Skeletal muscles are connected to our bones and work in opposing pairs, one muscle in the pair contracts while the other relaxes as in Figure 3-2, to create diverse body movements such as walking or picking up a coin.

The other two muscle groups are smooth muscles, found in the walls of internal body organs and the specialized muscle tissues of the heart. The Guide deals with only the skeletal muscle groups.

Muscles are made up of many strands of tissue called *fascicles*. You've probably noticed them when slicing into red meat or poultry.

Figure 3-2.
Forearm raised.

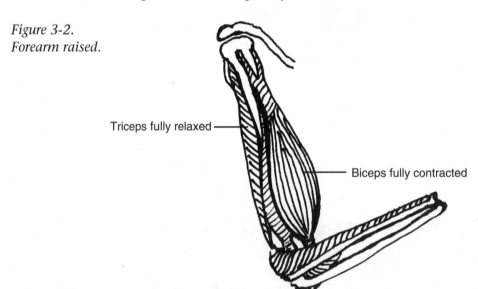

Triceps fully relaxed

Biceps fully contracted

Each fascicle is made up of bundles of muscle fibers called fasciculi and each fiber is constructed of, ready for this, tens of thousands of *myofibrils*. Myofibrils are thread-like and have the ability to contract, relax, and lengthen. I'm not quite done with the myo-fibrils yet, because they in turn are made up of millions of bands called *sarcomers*, with each sarcomer made up of overlapping thick and thin *myofilaments*. Almost done, hold on. The thick and thin myofilaments are comprised of contractile proteins.

Okay, so what does all this mean to you? Did you think just taking a step was simple? I told you muscles were like Congress—it's amazing we can even move our fingertips. Here's what happens when you want to cause a muscle to work; it's almost as complicated as passing a bill:

1. When you decide to move, the muscle is contacted by a nerve, which sends an electrical signal deep inside the muscle fibers.

2. This signal stimulates the flow of calcium, which causes the thick and thin myofilaments to slide across each other.

3. As this occurs, the sarcomers shorten, which generates force.

4. When billions of these sarcomers shorten in the muscle at one time, the entire muscle fiber contracts. But remember, this is only one very small fiber of the muscle.

5. If a weak contraction is required to do the task at hand, only a limited number of fibers will be called on to contract.

6. If you need strength, this requires a contraction of many more muscle fibers. The more strength required, the more fibers contract.

Muscles are attached to bones by tendons. Using the femur as an example, the muscles connected to it are connected both at the hip and knee. Now it starts to make sense why a flexibility problem in one area can also cause a problem in another area. Especially when you understand that as muscles are used they consume their fuel and fatigue, which means they shorten.

Here's where stretching comes in. When the muscle fatigues and shortens, the bands of thick and thin myofilaments that slid across each other are overlapped more than they should be, shortening the muscle. When you stretch the muscle, the amount of overlap decreases, allowing the muscle to lengthen. As you stretch, any disorganized fibers are realigned in the direction of the tension.

Chris's Concerns

I'm not a doctor and I don't play one on TV. However, throughout this Guide I want to be sure you understand that stretching can only help when a muscle is causing a problem and needs to be re-educated and its range of motion increased. Pain and injuries need to be immediately evaluated by a physician.

Joints: The Judiciary

I promise this is the last of my government analogies. In government, the Judiciary decides if laws or situations that arise are in line with the intent of the Constitution. Well, the joints in our body, are the ultimate judge if something violates the Constitution of Flexibility.

Since this Guide deals with stretching and flexibility, I won't get into the joints that are not designed for movement, but if you're playing Scrabble and looking for a 12-letter word starting with S, try "synarthroses."

Earlier I told you the location where two bones come together is called a joint. In the case of movable joints like hips and shoulders, the bones need a little cushioning and fluid to help the muscles move them smoothly. Bones in movable joints are covered by a smooth layer of *cartilage,* for cushioning and protective purposes and lubricated by thick fluid called *synovial fluid.* The fluid is produced in a sac located between the bones known as *bursae.* You may have heard of or even had a case of *bursitis,* a fairly common and painful condition of movable joints, caused by an inflammation of the bursae.

There are several types of moveable joints, as described in the following table.

Type of Joint	Movement	Examples
Ball and socket joints	Free movement in all directions	Hip, shoulder (see Figure 3-3)
Hinge joints	Elbows, knees, fingers	Moves in one plane only
Pivot joints	Permits rotation only	Between the first two neck vertebrae*
Gliding joints	Surfaces of bones move a short distance over each other	Some bones of the wrist and ankle

*Your head rotates from side to side using this type of joint, located between your first and second vertebrae.

The table illustrates all joints are not alike. Even similar joints differ in the amount of movement they allow. For instance, even though the hip and shoulder both have ball-and-socket–type joints, the shallowness of the shoulder socket allows more motion than the deeper-set socket of the hip.

Mr. Stretch Explains
Range of motion is a way of measuring the flexibility of the joint. If you can't move around the joint in a free, unobstructed manner, you have a limited range of motion and have a feeling of tightness. Healthy stretching is designed to restore the normally expected range of motion.

As you have learned, muscles are connected to the bones across the joints and move them by a series of contractions and re-lengthening by opposite muscle groups. Each type of joint allows a specific motion to take place. However, if a muscle group is fatigued or does not know it's supposed to be at a certain length, the *range of motion* for that joint will be limited.

In our first chapter, I used the Tin Man in *The Wizard of Oz* as an example of how we're not supposed to move. As you can see, we don't move in a straight line but instead we rotate. If you're sitting reading this, rotate your body around. The same thing takes place when you turn the page. Hold your wrist with your other hand and rotate it in various directions and see how it moves rotationally.

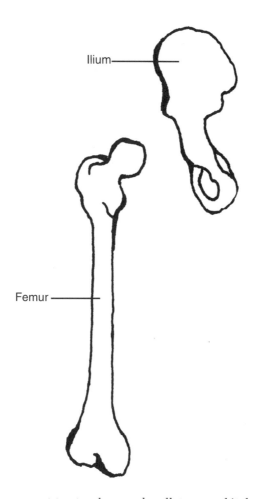

Figure 3-3. Hip ball and socket joint.

Ilium

Femur

Let's say you want to stand up and walk to your kitchen to get a drink. Here's what happens:

1. As you sit up, your hip joints have to rotate to propel you to stand.

2. Your knee joint slightly rotates along with your ankle joint as you stand up.

3. As you're beginning to stand, the pelvis rotates around the hip joints to achieve a balanced standing position.

4. The hips, knees, and ankles all rotate to propel you forward as the body has to constantly move, adjust, and balance itself through the joints to keep you on your feet.

5. Your arms rotate around their joints for added balance.

The flexibility self-test in Chapter 1 gave you an idea of your range of motion in the various joints. Healthy stretching will improve and then maintain that motion by educating your muscles so you can have the best range of motion possible through your joints.

If Your Body Is a Computer, Some Muscles May Have a "Virus"

I promised no more government analogies, so let's turn to computers instead. If you have a computer, you're well aware of hidden problems called viruses. Well, you may have some hidden problems in your body and, most likely, they've disguised themselves. It's not a virus but muscles that may be turned off or on vacation, not doing their jobs.

Compensating for the Vacationing Muscle

Compensating can be a fairly common occurrence and will help you understand whenever I refer to re-educating muscles.

In the injury section of Chapter 2, I explained how muscles, in order to protect themselves, shorten to avoid further damage. To be clear on this, shorten is not the same as contraction, which generates the powerful source of movement.

The same thing applies if you're in the "sitter" category and decide to go running. Some of the muscles you need to run with have adjusted themselves to the shorter length needed to comfortably accommodate your mostly sitting lifestyle.

So, like a computer virus, these are some hidden problems that can cause further problems. Your muscles don't mean to be a problem, they just don't know any better. Actually, they are very cooperative and doing what is supposedly in your best interest, only it's not.

You Heard What?

If you think kids are more flexible than adults, that's a misconception. You may think adolescents possess incredible flexibility when you see the way they run around, but some of their muscles may also be on vacation. This can cause some limited flexibility in their joints, just as in your case. The adolescent athletes I work with need to stretch to educate their muscles too.

Chapter 17 is all about children. You'll be surprised to learn that some of the injuries they develop later in life are a result of flexibility problems they have today.

These muscles are on vacation, making some other muscle group pick up the slack for the work they're not performing. As we now know, the body makes compensations to accommodate what you want to do, sometimes to the detriment of other muscles, resulting in a lack of flexibility and potential injury.

Oh, and if you ask a vacationing muscle to do something it's not prepared for or used to doing—watch out! Deciding to run, for example, when you sit most of the time is like someone waking you up in the middle of the night by throwing ice water on your face. You'd protest too. Just as a hidden computer virus shuts down a computer, these vacationing muscles can shut your flexibility down and affect the quality of your life.

Healthy Stretching Sends the Muscle a Wake-Up Call

When I refer to re-educating the muscle with healthy stretching here's what happens. As the muscle is gently stretched and the joint regains its intended flexibility, the muscle sends a signal alerting the brain to the fact that the muscle can work at this level. It's a complete re-education process as the muscle proves to the brain it can perform at the levels expected of it. The muscle shows it can respond to what it may be asked to do. That's why if you're a "sitter," but you like to run sometimes, keeping your muscles educated and stretched during the week will keep them ready to respond to the demands of running.

The flexibility of the stretched-out muscle allows it to develop more power as it contracts. Longer length provides more movement in its contraction. Lots of people have incredible strength in their muscles that can't be utilized because of the lack of flexibility. So stretching will help you get stronger as you tap into your muscles' potential. You're not creating strength, you're just tapping into what's potentially there.

This is the reason for some of the success attained by the professional athletes I stretch. Healthy stretching unlocks this hidden potential by returning the muscle to its proper length, allowing it to raise performance levels to new heights. Professional athletes may know how to use their body better than the average person, but they have many of the same flexibility problems you might have. Look at this as a hidden, untapped gold mine you'd like to discover, and it's there just waiting to be found.

The Least You Need to Know

➤ Bones are the load-bearing structure of the body.

➤ Muscles provide movement by contracting.

➤ A joint is the meeting location for two bones.

➤ Different types of joints allow the bones to rotate in specific movements.

➤ Some muscles may not be working to their full potential.

➤ Healthy stretching re-educates the muscle to be prepared for your demands.

41

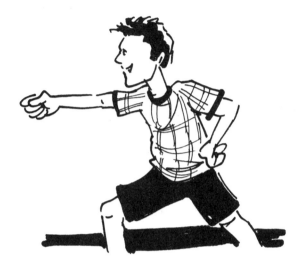

Chapter 4

Okay, Gang, Here's What Healthy Stretching Will Do for You

In This Chapter

➤ Healthy stretching can give you more energy

➤ Raise your performance levels in sports, even if you're an amateur

➤ How to start and benefit from the healthy stretching technique

➤ Stretching tips to maximize your results

➤ Connect some stretches together to increase your range of motion

Are you ready to increase your energy to get more from life? Are you ready to stimulate your muscles, making them easier to move? Then you're just about ready to begin enjoying *Mr. Stretch's flexibility technique of healthy stretching*. Notice I didn't say "routine" and I never mentioned "workout."

Both those terms have the negative connotation that you'll be spending lots of time doing laborious exercises, when the opposite is true. Glance ahead in the Guide and see how Mr. Stretch's technique blends into your daily life. Of course, there's no law forbidding you to do more if you like. A muscle already stretched to maximum does not need to be stretched beyond its normal length, just maintained, so the more flexible you become, the less time you need to spend stretching.

Before we start, here are some of the ways my healthy stretching technique works for professional athletes and how it will work for you:

➤ Golfers will swing with less effort, increasing clubhead speed, and be more consistent with distance and accuracy.

➤ Tennis players will increase foot speed and agility as well as creating better upper-body rotation.

➤ Basketball players can reduce lower-back discomfort, increase vertical leap, and improve lateral quickness.

➤ In-line skaters can improve reaction time and have better balance while increasing length of stride.

➤ Hardball and softball pitchers throw 3–5 mph faster with more control.

➤ Athletes can throw, run, jump, and swing to their full potential.

➤ The potential for injuries will be reduced as the muscles are conditioned to operate within their full range of motion.

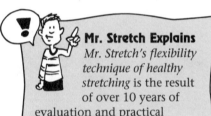

Mr. Stretch Explains

Mr. Stretch's flexibility technique of healthy stretching is the result of over 10 years of evaluation and practical application in the area of injury prevention and performance enhancement. The technique enables athletes to perform at maximum levels with better body awareness while minimizing risk of injury.

Stretching Strategies

Part 4 of the Guide features many of the sports you may participate in. The same stretches I use with the pros are featured to help you get the most from your game and potentially limit the risk of injury.

You may not be a professional athlete, but still want to get the best possible results from your efforts. Chances are you're taking lessons that only seem to help when the instructor is working with you. When you're on your own, however, the "magic" seems to disappear.

Let's use golf as an example of what I mean. Your golf pro most likely worked with you on posture and position. Pros will continuously correct these faults as they creep back during the lesson. As a result, you'll hit higher percentages of better shots while the pro is with you during the lesson.

On your own, without a pro to keep correcting you, your body slowly retreats back into the muscle comfort zone or flexibility range. Consequently, you'll revert back to your old game. Your pro was asking you to make changes your muscles could not comfortably maintain. In other words, the new swing is not right for your body in its present limited flexibility shape.

My healthy stretching technique will allow you to re-educate your muscles to take advantage of the pro's instruction, just as golfer Nick Price did with his instructor David Leadbetter. My stretching Nick allowed him to comfortably make and maintain the swing changes Leadbetter was asking for. Nick's string of victories since then proves he made the changes successfully. Pro athletes may have more skills at their command than the average person, but still have the same flexibility problems.

Together We've Identified Your Problems

Chapter 1 provided the opportunity to test your flexibility and range of motion. Chapter 2 showed how lifestyle and history have played a role. So by now you have a pretty good idea where your flexibility problems are and the categories you're in.

For instance, if you're in the "sitter" category, you've learned that your limited flexibility requires that certain muscle groups need to be re-educated as you stretch them out to their proper functioning length. If you're in the "stander" category, you now understand fatigued muscles need to be stretched out to keep supporting your weight comfortably. With this new awareness, the ability to target in on your own flexibility problems will be easier.

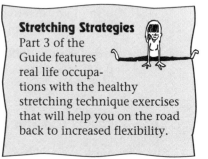

Stretching Strategies
Part 3 of the Guide features real life occupations with the healthy stretching technique exercises that will help you on the road back to increased flexibility.

If You're Having Pain, You Should See a Doctor

I can't emphasize enough that if you're experiencing real pain in your muscles or joints, go to your doctor and have it checked out before beginning the stretches. That's only common sense. We can work together improving the quality of your life by increasing your flexibility, but pain is something you need to have checked. If you have a history of back problems, I also suggest consulting your doctor before starting any of the healthy stretching technique exercises.

So, Mr. Stretch, How Do I Start?

That depends on your current level of flexibility based on the self-test. Here's my suggestion list to help get you started:

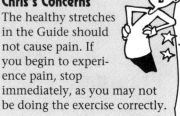

Chris's Concerns
The healthy stretches in the Guide should not cause pain. If you begin to experience pain, stop immediately, as you may not be doing the exercise correctly.

1. For the first week, you may want to start slowly with the healthy stretches in Part 2.

2. Start your day with The Wake-Up Wonders in Chapter 5. Some of them you can even do in bed.

3. About two hours before going to bed, do the Nightcaps in Chapter 7. I know you'll really enjoy doing these with a partner.

4. If you need a boost of energy during the day, try some stretches from Chapter 6, especially the Spark Ignitors.

5. Follow the Stretching Strategies sidebars throughout the Guide for suggestions on increasing your range of motion for your less flexible areas.

Feeling better right from the start is what usually happens, so you'll probably want to do more. Since I'm your own stretching coach, please follow the photos and do the stretches exactly the way we demonstrate them. I want you to get the maximum benefit from this Guide.

As you start feeling the benefits of the healthy stretches in Part 2, find your category in Part 3. It's not unusual to fit into several categories. For instance an "office worker" could also be a "captured commuter." It's okay to do the healthy stretches for both.

Regardless of your current flexibility, always do the healthy stretches demonstrated in Part 4, the sports section, before and after you participate.

You Heard What?

If you're like most people, you think stretching only needs to be done before participating in your favorite sport. That's a misconception. Muscles become fatigued and shorten *after* they've been used. Re-educate muscles back to their proper length by stretching immediately after you're done playing. Conveniently, the healthy stretches demonstrated in the sports section can be done right where you are. For instance, before and after golf stretches can be done using a golf cart or bench. Regardless of the sport, always stretch after participating to maintain your flexibility.

Another good idea is to take the flexibility test once a month to evaluate the range of motion for the various joints. The test will always point you in the right direction to maintain your flexibility with healthy stretching for your tight muscles.

Blend Healthy Stretching With Other Exercise Programs

Earlier in the Guide I mentioned there are many more people who hate to exercise than those who enjoy it. Most of us wish we could achieve the results rather than do the exercise. However, if you're dedicated to really improving overall body tone and your cardiovascular system, most likely you're already participating in a program of regular exercise. It could be strength training with weights, aerobics, or making the circuit of the machines at your health club.

Just like the professional athletes I work with daily, you need to include healthy stretching as part of your current exercise program. If strength or machine circuit training is your main focus, I suggest stretching immediately before and after strengthening. Think of it this way: Stretch before you strengthen and stretch after you strengthen. This maintains your full range of motion for the muscle groups.

You're Almost Ready to Start: Some More Important Tips

As your personal healthy stretching coach, I want to make sure you really understand how to correctly do the stretches in the Guide. Here's a short list of additional suggestions I want you to follow:

1. Follow the photos and descriptions of each healthy stretch. Take your time and check your positions for maximum effect.

2. As you reach each stretching position, use *the 15-second hold*.

3. The squeaking wheel gets more grease.

4. Connect your stretches to achieve flexibility. Several joints may need to be stretched to solve flexibility problems.

The first point is easy to understand and, since I know you're all ready to get started, I won't dwell on it except to say, please follow the directions. The next three sections explain what I mean by the other tips.

The 15-Second Hold: 15 Seconds That Can Change Your Life

I know you really want healthy stretching to improve your life, so I'm sure you'll follow my coaching and each photo to ease yourself into the proper stretching position. What's the next step once you've reached it?

Let's use a hip stretching exercise as an example. You're familiar with this one since it was part of the hip flexibility test in Chapter 1. This healthy stretch starts by having you sit in a straight-back chair, with one leg crossed so that the ankle is resting on the opposite thigh. Remember when I asked you how high your knee was up in the air?

To perform this stretch, you need to gently push down on the knee until you feel resistance. At this point you do *the 15-second hold*, continuing to press down for 15 seconds. Then relax the leg and change sides.

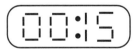

Figure 4-1. Fifteen seconds on your digital watch.

Why hold the stretching position for 15 seconds? Remember we're trying to re-educate your muscle back to the longer length that provides the increased range of motion and flexibility you need. Holding a muscle in a stretched position, even if it's only a slight stretch to begin with, allows the muscle to become accustomed to the new length. When it's not used to being at this length it is not happy, so the muscle signals the brain that it feels as if it is being stretched for too long a time.

As I developed my healthy stretching technique, I found the ideal time for holding the muscle, re-educating it to a longer length, is 15 seconds. As you hold the healthy stretch, the muscle begins to understand it can function at this new length and reduces its signaling.

Figure 4-2. Fifteen seconds on a stopwatch.

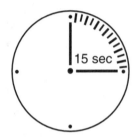

15 sec

Each time you stretch the muscle to the point where you encounter resistance and then push gently, it trains your *stretch receptors,* responsible for signaling, allowing the muscle to lengthen. That's why these healthy stretches are not very time-consuming. Why spend a lot of time when each stretch is effective in 15 seconds? To work best, I want you to repeat the stretch two or three times, depending on which side is the *squeaking wheel.*

The Squeaking Wheel Gets More Grease

As the pioneers trekked westward, they were ever vigilant to a wagon breaking down if a wheel came off. Squeaking was an indication a wheel was beginning to have a problem and needed to be taken care of. The squeaking wheel got the grease because it needed it more than the other three.

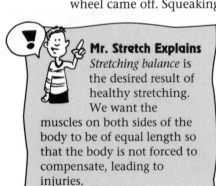

Mr. Stretch Explains
Stretching balance is the desired result of healthy stretching. We want the muscles on both sides of the body to be of equal length so that the body is not forced to compensate, leading to injuries.

Now, I'm not insinuating that your body is like a pioneer's Conestoga wagon, with your wheels so inflexible that they're squeaking like crazy. Or are they? The analogy helps put the squeaking-wheel-gets-more-grease saying into a stretching perspective. Let's use the same hip stretching exercise as an example.

As you did this stretching test, most likely one knee was higher than the other after you placed opposite ankles on your thighs. That side is the one we want to not only stretch

48

but also bring into *stretching balance* with the other side. In our analogy, the higher knee is the *squeaking wheel*.

When we just discussed the 15 seconds, I suggested two or three repetitions of each stretch, depending on which side was the squeaking wheel. Repeat the stretch three times for the stiffer side and only once or twice for the more flexible side in order to achieve flexibility balance.

An imbalance causes body compensations that have a huge effect. Take walking, for example. If you walk with one of your feet pointed out, a flexibility problem that most likely can be attributed to hip tightness, your ankle and knee are also affected. It doesn't do an awful lot of good for your shoe's outside heel either; it wears out faster.

Connect Your Stretches: Several Areas May Need to Be Re-Educated

Remember the old camp song that goes "The hip bone's connected to the thighbone, the thighbone's connected to the shinbone?" Well, it's true. It's especially true with flexibility problems. Here's a stretching table to illustrate areas you need to stretch for various flexibility problems.

Flexibility Problem	Areas That Should Be Stretched
Knees	Knees, hips, thighs, ankles
Ankles	Ankles, knees
Lower back	Lower back, hips, knees, ankles
Shoulder	Shoulder, neck, elbow
Neck	Neck, shoulder

I know you're ready to get started and start reaping the benefits of the healthy stretching technique. The one last thing I want to emphasize is—have fun with this technique. It's not work, it's freedom.

The Least You Need to Know

➤ Healthy stretching will help you increase your energy.

➤ Healthy stretching will stimulate your muscles, making them easier to move.

➤ If you're having pain in your muscles or joints, see a doctor before doing the stretches.

➤ Hold the stretch for 15 seconds and do one more repetition for the stiffer side.

➤ Connect several area stretches together to achieve flexibility.

Part 2
Stretch the Day: Mr. Stretch's Pick-and-Choose Menu

As the tensions of the day begin setting in and your energy starts to wane, I'll be there with the solution. As your new 24-hour-a-day flexibility coach, I have some healthy stretches you can blend into your life without taking lots of time. We'll even start before you get out of bed.

As the day draws to a close, you'll be able to do some healthy stretches with a partner that will ease away all the tightness and tensions from your busy day.

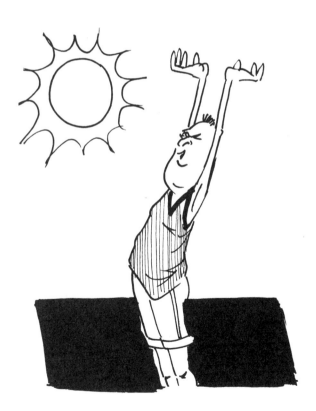

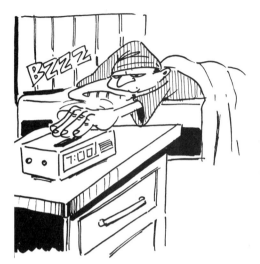

Chapter 5

Good Morning:
The Wake-Up
Wonders

In This Chapter

➤ Wake up your body before you get out of bed

➤ Healthy stretches invented by your dog or cat

➤ Facing the day

➤ How to use your towel for stretching

➤ Mr. Stretch helps you develop morning power

As the birds softly chirp, beginning their daily celebration of a new day, one eye slowly blinks open. The faint aroma of freshly brewed coffee wafts up the stairs into your bedroom. You wrap the blanket around yourself, trying to savor the last few precious quiet moments before the hectic pace of the day begins.

You're aware of soft footsteps coming up the stairs. The doorknob creaks almost imperceptibly, yet you hear it, as the door slowly opens. Perhaps you drifted back to sleep and thought these were imagined sounds from a last bit of dreaming. Then you hear me softly whisper in your ear: "Time to do your Wake-Up Wonders." Hey, I take my new job as your personal healthy stretching coach seriously.

Yawn Busters—Not Even Out of Bed and You're Already Stretching

Our first group of stretches together and you don't even have to get out of bed. Am I a nice guy or what? Seriously, the stretches I call the Yawn Busters are really a healthy way to start the day. You don't have to rush into them; just do them slowly, feeling the benefits immediately.

Undercover Body Stretch

When you slept, your blood pooled to an even level. Your body was probably in a fetal position most of the night, compressed. You may have been under some tension the day before so your body may still be a little tense. The body stretch allows you to stretch everything out.

Photo 5-1 (Left). Start by lying with your hands relaxed by your sides. Photo 5-2 (Right). Put your hands together, reaching up as far as you can, then push your toes as far down as you can.

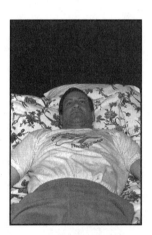 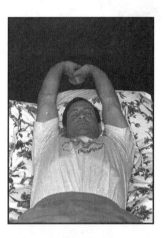

Hold for 15 seconds. Your whole spine gets stretched, allowing you to feel the length of your body.

Chris's Concerns

If you have a water-bed, you may find it a little more difficult to do this healthy stretch. Give it a try, but if you don't have the proper support, the stretch can still be done on the floor of your room.

Morning Hamstring Stretch

I think it's a good idea for you to get your legs moving before getting out of bed. Since supporting your weight all day is one of their job descriptions, they'll appreciate a gentle wake-up call. This healthy stretch concentrates on your *hamstring muscles,* located in the back of your leg. Sorry, but you have to get out from under the covers.

Your hips will also start to wake up and move. The stretch allows each side to move independently as you stretch side to side. I'd like you to do this two times, for each side, being sure to hold the raised position for 15 seconds as you educate the muscles.

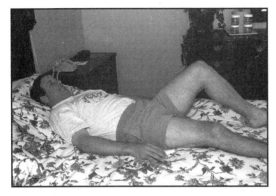

Photo 5-3. Remain relaxed, lying on the bed, and gently slide your left foot back, keeping it in contact with the bed as you raise one knee. Keep your hands by your side and the other leg straight.

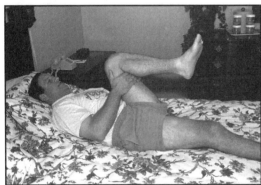

Photo 5-4. Reach up and grab behind your left knee with both hands. Gently pull your knee toward your chest, stopping when you start to feel some resistance (tightness or tension). You should feel a slight stretching of your hamstring.

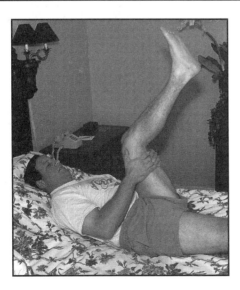

Photo 5-5. Slowly raise your left foot up. You don't have to straighten your leg, just raise it up enough to develop a stretching feeling in your hamstring. The act of moving your foot up is putting tension on the hamstring, stretching it. Hold in this position for 15 seconds. Relax your body back into the starting position, and repeat with the right leg.

Two Knees to the Chin

You'll really start feeling good with this healthy stretch. It's a great way to provide some additional stretch to the hamstrings and derrière as you start to stretch the lower back. Repeat this stretch twice, holding for 15 seconds.

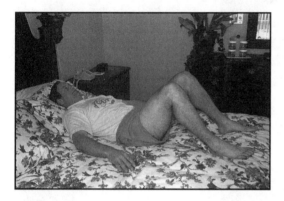

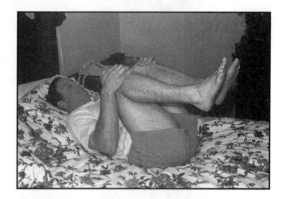

Photo 5-6. Still lying relaxed on your bed, hands to your side, slide both feet back, raising both knees.

Photo 5-7. Reach up, gently, with both hands as the left hand grabs the left knee and the right hand grabs the right knee. Pull your knees toward your chest.

Two Knees to the Side

Now we want to let your *torso muscles* in the midsection of your body know it's time to wake up. This healthy stretch of the torso muscles, those in the area we all like to call the stomach and those in the lower back, require some morning education dealing with rotation. Repeat this healthy stretch two times, holding for 15 seconds.

Photo 5-8. Begin from the same knees-up starting position, but this time, keep both knees together.

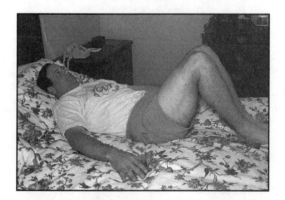

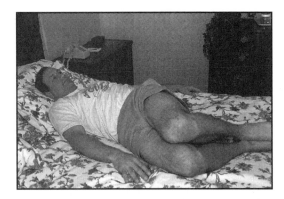

Photo 5-9. Keeping your knees together, roll to one side keeping both shoulders touching the bed. Roll only as far as you can, making sure you keep your knees together. If your knees can't touch the bed, don't worry. All I want you to do is wake up the torso muscles, not stretch them.

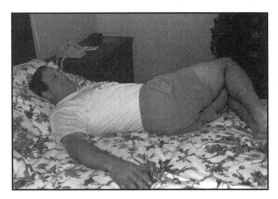

Photo 5-10. Now roll to the other side, keeping your shoulders in contact with the bed and your knees together. As you repeat this stretch, try to feel that you get your knees a little closer to the bed each time, if you're not flexible enough to actually touch it.

Mr. Stretch's Healthy Way to Get Out of Bed

I'm pleased with your progress so far. You should be feeling pretty good, lying in bed, with muscles already awake and ready to get the day started. You may be feeling so good you want to jump out of bed, but please don't. Lots of people actually start the day with muscle injuries caused by twisting themselves and contorting their bodies just with the simple act of getting out of bed. Here's a suggestion list for a healthy way to get up:

➤ Start by rolling on your side facing the edge of the bed.

➤ Bend your knees 90 degrees to your waist. If we had a skycam looking down, you would be in a "Z" position.

➤ Next, let your feet go off the edge of the bed.

➤ Using a hand as leverage, push yourself up to a sitting position.

➤ Now stand up.

This healthy way to get out of bed avoids stress on various muscle groups. Stress can cause muscle damage.

The Floor Four: Learning From Your Dog or Cat

Whenever your dog or cat wakes up from a nap, the first thing they do is stretch. It's a natural instinct. This next group of healthy stretches helps get your spinal fluid moving. I think the spine, being your lifeline, is the most important part of your body.

Back Arch

You could call this the "cat and dog stretch," since you'll always see them do these several times a day. Repeat this series of movements five times holding five or six seconds in each position.

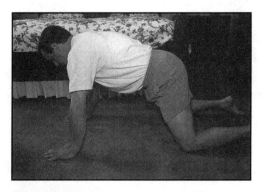

Photo 5-11. Begin by getting on your hands and knees, keeping your back straight.

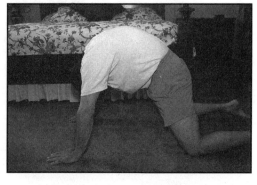

Photo 5-12. I haven't lost my head. I've just tucked my chin toward my chest as I tilt my back and pelvis up forming an arch, creating a rounded look. Hold this position for five or six seconds.

Photo 5-13. Reverse everything by raising your chin from your chest, bringing your head up as you drop your pelvis down, forming a very slight "U" shape. Hold for five or six seconds and repeat the movements.

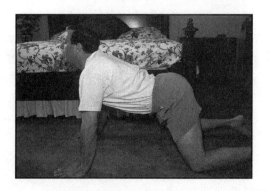

You Heard What?

If you think jumping out of bed is the best way to start the day, you'd be wrong. Along with the stress you put on your muscles, you can feel light-headed caused by the fact that your blood pressure hasn't stabilized itself. Just because you're lying in bed, maybe even watching television, doesn't mean your body knows it's awake. The muscles of the body have to start moving as they become educated to the fact they're awake.

Praying Stretch

My friend Steve Hosid, this Guide's co-author, has two Borzoi hounds that love this stretch. They run at 42 mph so you know they're flexible. It's an easy exercise to do first thing in the morning, creating movement in several joints at the same time. The sections of your body benefiting from this healthy stretch are the shoulders, arms, back, hips, and knees. Repeat three times, holding for 15 seconds.

In this stretch, you're rotating on your hip and shoulder joints as you try to sit back on your heels.

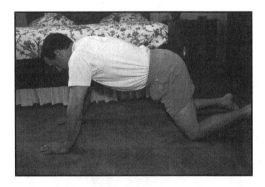

Photo 5-14. Begin this healthy stretch by getting on your hands and knees, keeping your back straight.

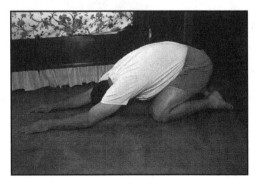

Photo 5-15. Keeping your hands in the same position, slide back on your knees, trying to touch your derrière to your heels.

59

Torso Press Up

Now we want to stretch the front of your torso. It's another way to arch your back. Only go part-way up if you feel resistance in your stomach or lower back. You can go all the way up to the arched advanced position if you don't feel resistance. Repeat this stretch three times, holding the position in Photo 5-18 for 15 seconds.

Photo 5-16. Lay face down on the floor, hands next to your shoulders.

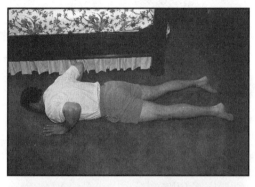

Photo 5-17. Press up slowly until you feel some resistance in your stomach or lower back. Hold for 15 seconds.

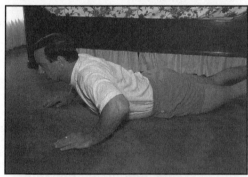

Photo 5-18. Advanced position. If you don't feel any pressure in your back, keep pressing up until you arch your back. Hold for 15 seconds.

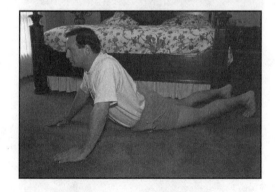

Walking Wake-Up Stretch

So far we've stretched several groups of muscles, preparing them for the day. Now we'll do a healthy stretch to educate the muscle groups needed for walking.

You should feel your right *quadriceps muscle,* located in the front of your thigh, gently stretch. I suggest you do three repetitions for each side and you'll walk to your car with newfound freedom.

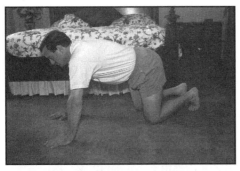

Photo 5-19. Back on your hands and knees again. Keep your back straight and in line with your head.

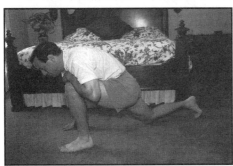

Photo 5-20. Bring your left foot up so it's now under your left knee. Place your left hand on your left knee.

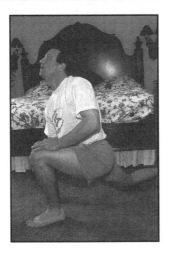

Photo 5-21. Press with your left hand as you pick your head, chin, and shoulders up. As you look toward the ceiling, your right knee remains on the ground. Hold for 15 seconds and repeat for the other leg.

Chris's Concerns

It's important you do the neck and chin exercises using your favorite cream or lotion. Doing the exercise on dry skin causes friction instead of the massaging action needed to achieve our goal. Always start at the bottom of the neck and go to the top, lift and start from the bottom of your neck again.

The Facial Two

Toning facial muscles can achieve a firmer chin and neckline. Your whole face can appear trimmer, toned, and perhaps younger-looking. This is not going to be a cosmetic cover-up; you're actually performing physical actions that work the muscle groups.

I'm not trying to sell you any special creams or lotions, so use any of your favorites, especially those that absorb into the skin and won't leave you with a greasy feeling. You don't have to go out and purchase any devices for this group either; everything you need is built into your hand.

Neck Toner

The *platysma muscle* is one muscle you really want to take care of. Banding and neck wrinkle lines are caused as this muscle loses its tone. So I suggest we keep it educated. Start by applying some of your favorite cream or lotion on your neck.

Repeat the movement shown in Photos 5-25 and 5-26 slowly and repeatedly for about 30 seconds.

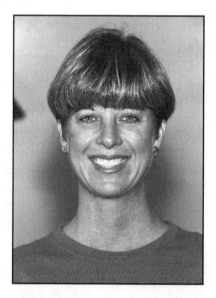

Photo 5-22. After you've applied the cream or lotion to your neck, smile and relax as you look at yourself in the mirror.

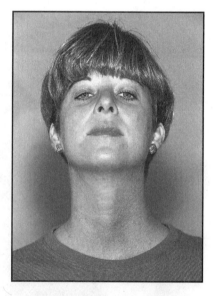

Photo 5-23. Raise your chin.

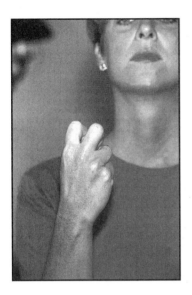

Photo 5-24. Bend your index finger (second finger) and middle finger so the two knuckles become rounded.

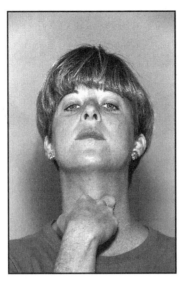

Photo 5-25. Place the knuckles on the bottom of your neck.

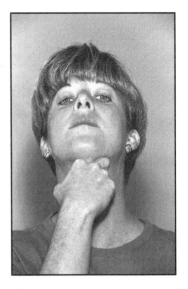

Photo 5-26. Gently but firmly move the knuckles upward until they reach your chin. You don't need to hold this position, just do it slowly and repeatedly for about 30 seconds.

Chin Chin

Now we want to tone the muscle group that works the chin. Those muscles need to be stimulated and re-educated too. After applying your favorite cream or lotion, use the knuckles again as you work on your chin line.

Never reverse the direction—always keep your knuckles moving upward. You don't have to hold the position, just slowly repeat the exercise for about 30 seconds for each side.

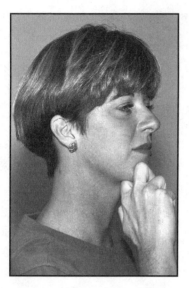

Photo 5-27. Start by placing
the knuckles on either side of
your chin, so you can press
your chin between them.

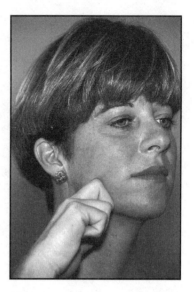

Photo 5-28. Move your knuckles
in an upward direction, keeping
the chin bone between them until
they are just below your ear.

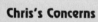

Mr. Stretch Explains
Feeling looser after
taking a shower is a
result of warmed
blood from the
surface being recirculated into
your body raising your core or
inner temperature. The
warmth produces suppleness
or pliability. Flexibility is a
result of the muscles moving.

Chris's Concerns
If you have a history of
back problems, do not
do the Front Bend. It's
also not recommended
for senior citizens.

Morning Power: After-Your-Shower Stimulators

Your muscles feel really loose after taking a shower, so how
about a few healthy stretches to send you off, full of energy
for the day ahead?

Front Bend

This stretch is an easy way to get your muscles to start
working. It's for the benefit of your lower back and sides
of your body, along with your hips and legs. This healthy
stretch allows you to work two muscle groups together: As
one stretches, the other relaxes. Repeat the stretch three
times, holding for 15 seconds with your head down and
15 seconds with your head up.

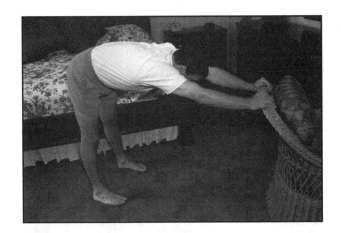

Photo 5-29. Stand with your feet shoulder-width apart. Bend over and grab the back of a chair, keeping your back straight and in line with your head.

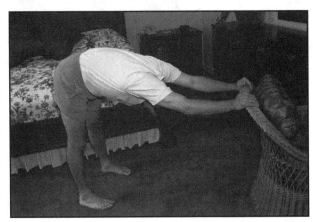

Photo 5-30. Push your head down as far as you can, stretching your spine. Hold for 15 seconds.

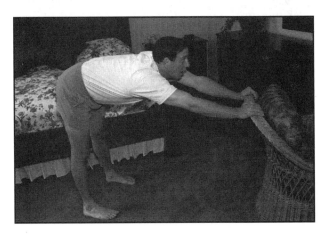

Photo 5-31. Pick your chin up, stretching all the muscles on the front of your body, as you contract the muscles of your spine. Hold for 15 seconds.

Bend Over Twist

You've probably been saying to yourself, "When's Chris going to get to my oblique muscles?" *Oblique muscles*, body rotators, are in the stomach and lower back area. I needed to have you stretch some other muscle groups first so we could progress safely to this very important group of muscles. Do two repetitions, holding each for 15 seconds.

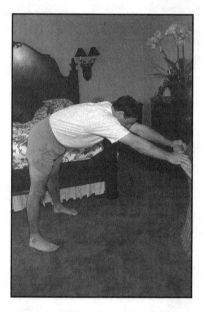

Photo 5-32. With your feet spread shoulder-width apart, bend over and grab the back of a chair.

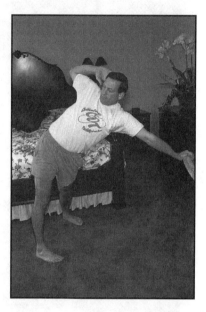

Photo 5-33. Take one hand, put it behind your head, and rotate that arm back leaving yourself balanced with the other hand on the chair.

Hold the position in Photo 5-33 for 15 seconds and then repeat the stretch, switching hands to stretch the other side. You should feel the twisting in your torso area. Feeling a stretching sensation in your chest area is a good indication of some inflexibility there.

Landing Eagle

We have so much to learn from our animal friends. We have to teach ourselves what they do naturally, by instinct. The Landing Eagle is a healthy stretch; and you'll find it a lot easier to do than its cousin the Spread Eagle. You'll be stretching the inner hamstring of one leg and the quadriceps of the other leg. I suggest you do this healthy stretch two times.

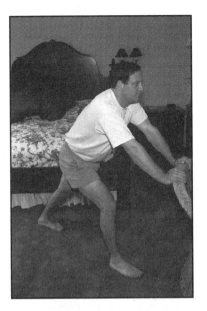

Photo 5-34. Stand with your feet slightly spread apart, pointing straight ahead. One knee is slightly bent, the other straight, as your hands hold onto the back of a chair.

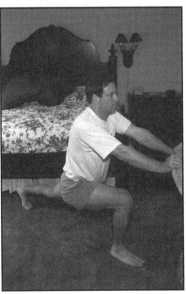

Photo 5-35. Lower your hips down so you form a 90-degree angle with your front knee. Hold for 15 seconds. Change legs and repeat by bending the opposite knee.

Wall Side Bend

Here we go using that fancy, expensive equipment again. I know you're so dedicated to feeling good you'll want to construct a wall to the exact specifications as mine. All kidding aside, one of the many benefits of healthy stretching is it can be done anywhere without having to lug anything along with you.

Now we need to stretch the upper arms, along with the area where your muscles are attached to the hips. This healthy stretch will educate your muscles and allow you to bend. Please do three repetitions, alternating for each side.

The body is stretching sideways, so you should feel the stretching on your side. Do not tilt to the front. Hold the position in Photo 5-37 for 15 seconds and repeat by changing positions for the other side.

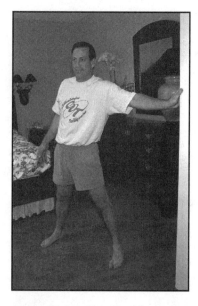

Photo 5-36. Stand with your feet slightly spread apart with one hand on a wall or door.

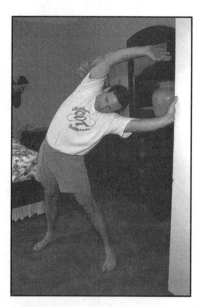

Photo 5-37. Take your opposite hand and raise it over your head, bringing it toward the wall as far as you can.

Towel Time: Don't Hang It Up to Dry Just Yet

You've started your day with some healthy stretches and a brisk shower. Don't hang up your towel to dry just yet! Let's use it to do some more healthy stretching. I know towels come in various sizes, but try to approximate the size you'll need from the photos.

Towel-Free Stretch

This is a very exhilarating stretch that you'll feel from the tips of your toes to your fingertips. I would like you to do it two or three times.

When you do this stretch, you should feel the stretch on the opposite side of the your body. Repeat for the other side, holding for 15 seconds.

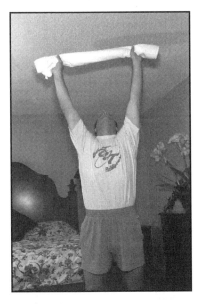

Photo 5-38. Hold a towel in both hands and raise it above your head as high as you can. You should feel a stretch pulling all over your body.

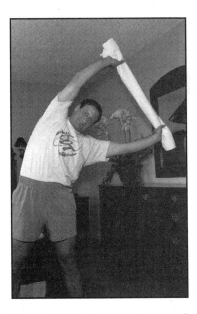

Photo 5-39. Keeping the towel tightly stretched between your hands, stretch to one side being careful to stay in the side-to-side stretch, not allowing your hands to move forward.

Horizontal Towel Stretch

This healthy stretch will really get your shoulders and upper back started for the day. How about doing this stretch two times, holding for 15 seconds?

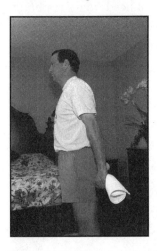

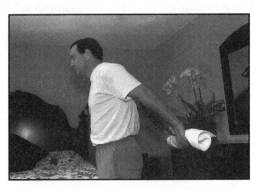

Photo 5-41. Lift your hands backwards away from your body as far as you can go.

Photo 5-40. Start by standing straight, your feet slightly spread apart. Hold the towel tightly stretched between your hands, shoulder-width apart.

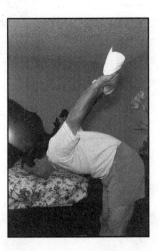

Photo 5-42. If you want to get more of a stretch, bend over and keep bringing your hands back. The farthest point you should go back would create an "L" shape between your arms and back.

Vertical Towel Stretch

The last healthy stretch to get you on your way is also done with the towel behind your back but this time it's going to be held vertically up and down. I want you to stretch your shoulders and the muscles in front and back of your arm to stretch out. It's a quick way to stretch several different muscle groups at the same time. Hold the position for 15 seconds and repeat three times for each side.

You'll feel the stretch in the front of your lower hand as well as the front of the lower hand's shoulder. The stretch can also be felt in the back of the arm. Hold the position in Photo 5-44 for 15 seconds and then repeat it, switching sides.

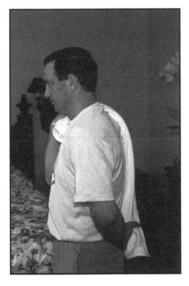

Photo 5-43. Throw the towel over your shoulder, grabbing it with one hand reaching back behind you while the other holds the top of the towel in front.

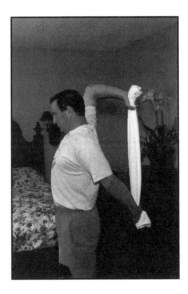

Photo 5-44. Keeping the towel tight, push it away from your body as your top hand pushes backward.

The Least You Need to Know

➤ Healthy stretching can begin under the covers of your bed.

➤ Just because you're awake doesn't mean your body is.

➤ The Yawn Busters will begin your healthy stretching day.

➤ Some of the best stretches mimic animals; they stretch by instinct.

➤ Healthy stretching can tone your neck and chin line.

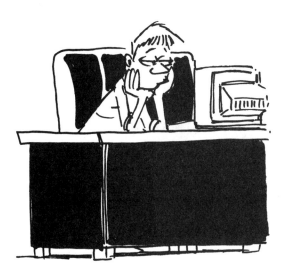

Chapter 6

Mid-Afternoon Energy Boosters

In This Chapter

➤ Healthy stretching—your Energy Foundation

➤ Forget the coffee—healthy stretching stimulates you faster

➤ Getting over the mid-afternoon slump and preparing for a great evening

➤ Tapping into energy reserves

The situation feels hopeless as ever so slowly your spent body drags itself toward the setting sun. Buzzards circle, anticipating a late afternoon snack. The furrows in your brow deepen, your eyes search for some glimpse of hope on the horizon.

Is that a mirage you see? At first it seems like a speck in the distance, but your heart beats faster as closer and closer it comes. Yes, my worn-out friend…Mr. Stretch is here to save you!

I may be a little over dramatic but, to some people, mid-afternoon can feel just like that scenario. Lunch was a few hours ago, they've been involved in other endeavors since early morning, and all their energy has been used up. The mind wanders, productivity suffers, but there is a way to build a *bridge of energy* to the evening. Can you guess what I'm about to say? Healthy stretching!

Mr. Stretch Explains
My experience shows healthy stretching is a *bridge of energy*, providing a means to convey you over the quagmire of the blahs. Stimulation of the muscles, as they're stretched, increases their blood supply and nutrition. This rejuvenates the body, providing you with energy.

Chris's Concerns
While the front squat is a great stretch to get your legs moving, don't try to get into the 90-degree knee angle if you hear your knees cracking as you lower into the squat.

So far, you've seen how easily stretching can be incorporated into your life without having to make major time commitments. You didn't think I'd leave you stranded in the toughest part of the day, did you? So, here are some mid-afternoon healthy stretches to get you revved up again. If the stretch directions suggest three repetitions but you're pressed for time, it's okay to do them once for each side.

Your Energy Foundation

To rebuild your energy levels and propel you merrily toward the evening, we need to start with a foundation. Most of the major muscle groups that move the body are located below your waist. If you're a "sitter," for example, you haven't been using your legs all day. This is a good time to get them going again. If you're on your legs all day, this is a good time to re-educate the muscles, bringing them back into balance, as we stretch out the fatigue.

Front Squat

Here's a healthy stretch to just get your lower body moving, setting the stage for the other Energy Foundation stretches. It's like a wake-up call, letting the lower body know it's going to be required to move.

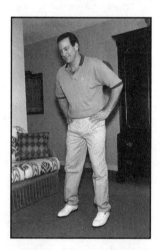

Photo 6-1. Stand with your hands on your hips, your knees slightly bent.

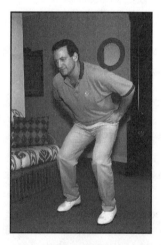

Photo 6-2. Lower down into a squat until you come to a point where you feel increased resistance. Your knees may ideally form a 90-degree angle, but don't force yourself into that position.

74

Consider the position in Photo 6-2 as your ultimate flexibility goal. Hold for three or four seconds, come back up and repeat five times.

Frog Squat

Whose legs are more powerful than a frog's? Comparing inches to feet, their vertical lift surpasses the jumping ability of an NBA superstar. You'll especially feel this stretch in your inner thigh.

I believe that most people's inner thigh muscles are weak and uneducated. Once you re-educate these muscles, they'll provide excellent support to your lower back while assisting other muscle groups in supporting your whole body.

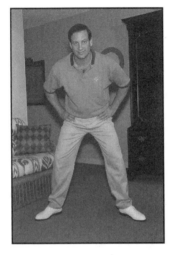

Photo 6-3. Start with your hands on your hips, knees slightly bent. Turn your feet slightly outwards.

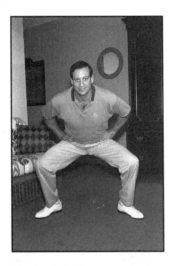

Photo 6-4. As you squat down, you'll feel the stretch on the inside of your thighs.

This muscle doesn't usually get used in other activities but it's a great supporter of other muscles. Now it can help some other tired muscles get through the rest of the day. Hold for three or four seconds, come up and repeat five times.

Chris's Concerns

If you start to feel any unusual pressure or discomfort in your lower back area stop at once. Recheck the directions for the Standing Calf stretch. If you again feel discomfort when you start the stretch, stop immediately. You may be stretching farther than your body can handle.

Squat Lunge

This healthy stretch re-educates the muscles on the inside of the stretched leg. Please hold the stretched position for 15 seconds and repeat three times, alternating legs.

You should still be facing forward as the lunge goes to the side as shown in Photo 6-6. The stretched out leg should be straight and feeling the stretch. Hold for 15 seconds. Do this stretch three times, alternating stretched sides.

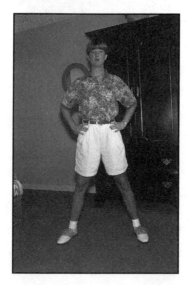

Photo 6-5. Stand with your feet wider than shoulder-width apart, hands on your hips.

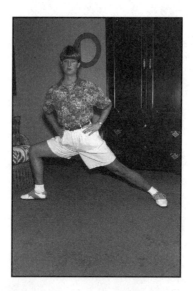

Photo 6-6. Keeping your body facing straight ahead, point one foot directly in the direction you want to lunge. Lower yourself so your knee goes over the ankle of the pointed foot.

Standing Calf Stretch

The key to this stretch is to try and keep your heel on the ground as you slowly and gently stretch the calf muscles, located in back of your lower leg. No special equipment is required and it can be done by anyone at any time.

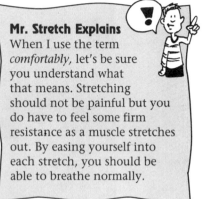

Mr. Stretch Explains
When I use the term *comfortably*, let's be sure you understand what that means. Stretching should not be painful but you do have to feel some firm resistance as a muscle stretches out. By easing yourself into each stretch, you should be able to breathe normally.

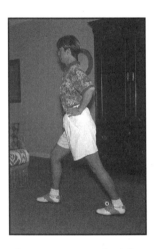

Photo 6-7. *Stand with your feet in line and split front to back a little wider than shoulder width. The incorrect tendency is to turn your back foot slightly out, so be sure they are in line.*

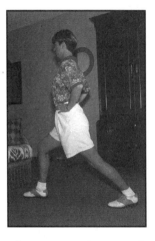

Photo 6-8. *Bring your front leg slightly and gently forward along with your hips, maintaining your body in an upright posture. Keep your back heel on the ground until you feel the calf muscle slightly stretching. Hold for 15 seconds, repeating two times for each side.*

Front Hip Flexor

Now that you've re-educated your leg muscles, let's start stretching the hip flexor muscles. As with all stretches, try to feel the stretch as you go through the various positions.

If you feel too much tightness to *comfortably* keep your stretched leg straight, it's okay to bend it. Hold for 15 seconds and repeat two or three times for each side. It's always a good idea to alternate sides for the stretches.

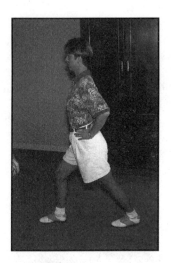

Photo 6-9. Begin this healthy stretch in the same starting position as the Standing Calf stretch with your feet in line, wider than shoulder width.

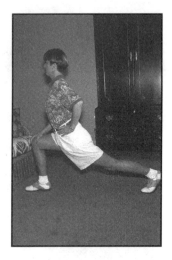

Photo 6-10. Slide your back foot backwards, lowering your hips until your front knee forms a 90-degree angle.

Energy Enhancers

This upper body group of healthy stretches further builds some flexibility started with the "Energy Foundation" stretches. As the muscles stretch out, the more energy you'll have. As I see it, energy starts in your lower body and flows to the upper body.

Hands Up

We need a simple stretch to start this group. While it may be simple, it begins the process. Healthy stretching doesn't shock the muscles but instead eases them into their proper lengths. Sometimes what appears simple is the foundation for region flexibility.

Feel this stretch all over your body. Go up on your toes if you like. Hold for 15 seconds and repeat two times. You'll find this stretch demonstrated in Photos 6-11 and 6-12.

Side Bend

Now let's start stretching your lower side muscles. These are your oblique muscle groups. Remember, ease yourself gently into the positions and feel the benefits of the stretching muscles. You may discover you haven't been able to move or be this flexible in years. See Photos 6-13 to 6-15.

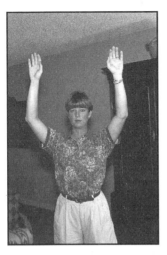

Photo 6-11. Put your hands above your head with your elbows bent so they're relaxed.

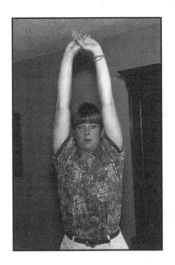

Photo 6-12. Put your hands together and push up straightening your elbows.

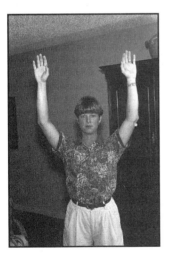

Photo 6-13. Start in the Hands Up position, elbows relaxed and bent slightly.

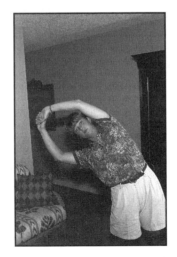

Photo 6-14. Bring your hands together and stretch as you did in Hands Up, feeling it all over your body. Now keeping that feeling, lean to one side. You should feel the extended side stretching. Hold for 15 seconds.

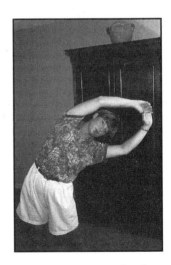

Photo 6-15. Now slowly go back to the straight position, continuing on until you lean on the other side. Hold for 15 seconds and do this healthy stretch two times.

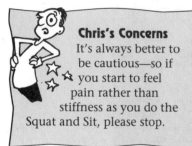

Chris's Concerns

It's always better to be cautious—so if you start to feel pain rather than stiffness as you do the Squat and Sit, please stop.

Squat and Sit

Do you have a desk or table available? You need a surface that's sturdy to hold onto as you stretch. You'll feel your lower back muscles and shoulders stretching.

As the knees reach a 90-degree angle as shown in Photo 6-17, your shoulders, torso, and lower back will be stretching. Hold for 15 seconds, then come back up and repeat two more times.

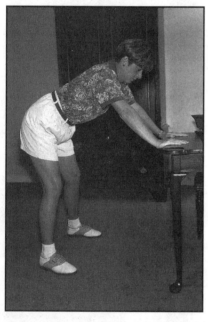

Photo 6-16. Stand facing the desk or table, feet spread about shoulder-width apart. Bend from the waist and grip the table.

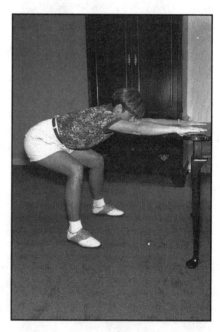

Photo 6-17. Sit back as you feel your shoulders straightening out. The feeling should be of pulling away from the table.

Afternoon Squat and Twist

We'll complete our upper body Energy Enhancers with one more healthy stretch. Your muscles are now stretched enough and are prepared to do this stretch.

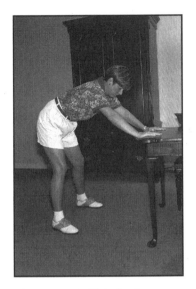 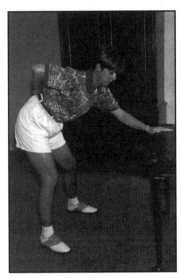 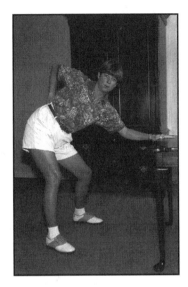

Photo 6-18. This is the same starting position for the Squat and Sit stretch, feet spread shoulder-width apart. Bend from the waist, keeping your back straight as you grab onto the desk or table.

Photo 6-19. Take one hand and put it behind your back.

Photo 6-20. Sit slightly back and twist the behind-your-back elbow and shoulder in a backwards rotational movement. Your shoulders should be almost perpendicular, almost like a right angle. You won't actually be able to reach 90 degrees, just use it as a guideline.

Tension Relaxers

All of us are pretty much aware that tension can be extremely detrimental to our health. It can cause high blood pressure, headaches, general malaise, and attitude problems. Tension is your physical response to emotional problems. You have tension if:

➤ Lincoln's neck on Mt. Rushmore is more flexible than yours.

➤ Someone walks up behind you, says hello, and you jump higher than Shaquille O'Neal.

➤ Steel company engineers ask if they can borrow the formula for your shoulders.

➤ You walk through airport security and your muscles trip the alarm.

We think of tension in different ways, but for the purposes of this Guide, let's consider what it does to your muscles. It tightens them, very often producing aches and pains. How many times a day do you rub your shoulders and neck thinking you can break the tension cycle? I believe doing some healthy stretching during the day helps stay ahead of the tension buildup. Here are some easy-to-do tension-relieving stretches to choose from.

Shoulder Shrug

Without your consciously knowing it, tension creeps into your shoulders. Along with outside emotional situations, just normal rotation and use of the muscles fatigues them, causing a feeling of tightness as they shorten. This relaxing stretch helps keep tension from settling in.

Hold for the position in Photo 6-22 for five seconds, relax, and repeat five times.

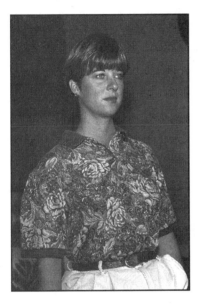

Photo 6-21. Relax and drop your shoulders down as far as you can, arms at your side.

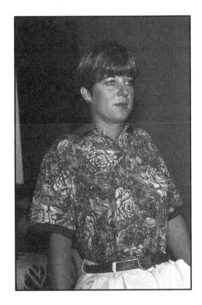

Photo 6-22. Raise your shoulders up and back pinching the muscles on the upper part of your shoulders with your neck, then pinching your shoulder blades together.

Seated Rowing Motion

This healthy stretch will help relieve some tension in your shoulders and neck. Hold the position in Photo 6-24 for five seconds. Then do the opposite, bringing your shoulder blades back trying to pinch them together, holding this position for five seconds. Please repeat five times and you'll be building a tension defense system.

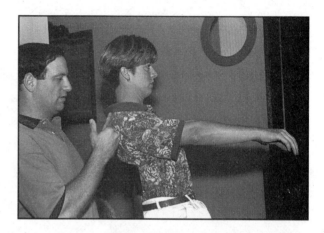

Photo 6-23. I have my hand on the back of Lisa's shoulder blades to illustrate the change in the shoulders for this healthy stretch. Raise your arms in front as you sit straight in a chair. Pinch your shoulder blades back while your arms stay straight.

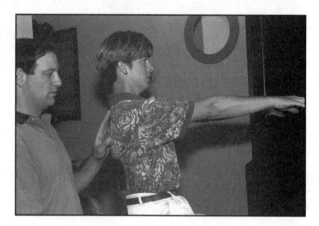

Photo 6-24. Try pushing your hands straight out in front as you feel the muscles between your shoulder blades stretch out.

Overhead Shrug

We continue stretching tension away by working our shoulders. I'm standing behind Lisa to show the difference in her shoulder height for the stretch.

Hold for five seconds before doing the reverse action of coming back down and lowering your shoulders as far as they can go with your arms still extended upwards. Hold this position for five seconds and repeat the entire stretch five times.

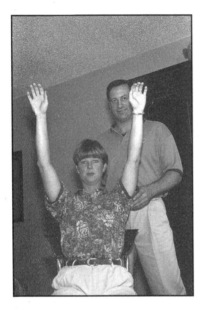

Photo 6-25. In the sitting position, Lisa puts her hands above her head, relaxed and loose with her elbows slightly bent.

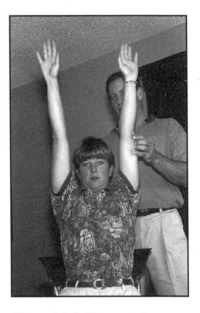

Photo 6-26. The stretch occurs as you straighten your arms and raise your shoulders up to your ears.

Shoulder Twist

If any tension is left, you'll twist it out of your muscles with this final Tension Relaxer healthy stretch.

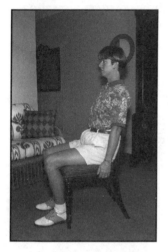

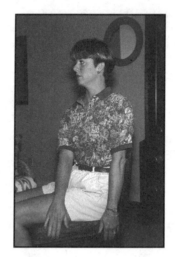

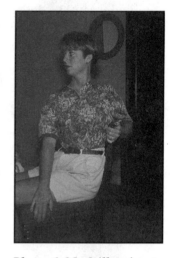

Photo 6-27. Begin this healthy stretch by sitting straight, but relaxed, in a chair. Keep your arms at your side.

Photo 6-28. Keeping your head and body facing forward, place both arms on one side of the chair.

Photo 6-29. Still trying to face forward, take one arm and move it back slowly so that it cradles the far back of the chair. Your shoulders should be perpendicular to your waist.

The movement back in Photo 6-29 is causing a twisting stretch of your shoulders helping keep tension away. Hold for 15 seconds and repeat, alternating shoulders, three times.

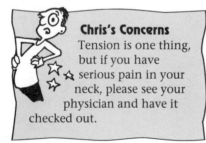

Chris's Concerns
Tension is one thing, but if you have serious pain in your neck, please see your physician and have it checked out.

Neck Minders

This is a case where if you really want to get rid of tension, stretch both the shoulders and the neck. We've just done the shoulders, so let's concentrate on a few neck stretches to maximize our Mid-Afternoon Energy Boosters.

Head Forward and Back Stretch

This is a good time of day to do some healthy, relaxing neck stretches. If you woke up with your neck feeling great and it's stiff as can be now, you have one incredibly stressful life. Take some time to pamper yourself. Start the soothing and relaxing process with some slow, deep breaths. Visualize the tension leaving your neck and shoulders as you exhale. Hey, I'm relaxing too much myself—we still have a few healthy neck stretches for you to try.

It's your choice to either stand or sit for this stretch, but please try to have the best posture either way. Close your eyes and try to focus in where you think the tension is. Relax and keep your chin up.

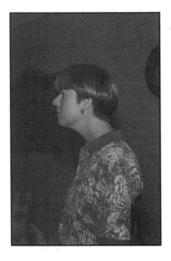

Photo 6-30. Push your chin slowly straight forward, keeping your shoulders in place. Perhaps think of yourself as a turtle, sticking its head out of a shell. You'll feel the stretch under your chin and the base of your neck. Hold for 15 seconds.

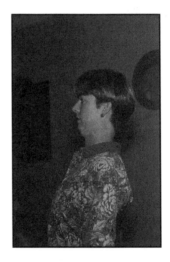

Photo 6-31. Now do the opposite as you bring your chin back as far as you can. Hold for 15 seconds. Repeat two or three times.

Ear to Shoulder

The average head weighs 12 pounds and is supported by the neck. The weight can fatigue the muscles, so let's help them out with some side-to-side stretches.

You Heard What?

When tension settles in, it's a common practice to quickly rotate the shoulders around and move the neck quickly in a circle. This is not correct; in fact, you may do some damage. Healthy stretching slowly stretches out the muscles holding them in the stretched position. The key is to do this regularly, keeping the muscles lengthened and tension-free.

Photo 6-32. Smile and relax, facing forward, standing or sitting with good posture.

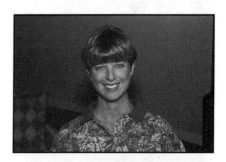

Photo 6-33. Keeping your head facing straight ahead, lean your head and try to touch your ear to your shoulder. Don't force it, you don't have to touch—just make it your goal. Hold for 15 seconds.

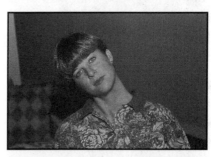

Photo 6-34. Reverse slowly moving your other ear toward the other shoulder trying, but not forcing, the two to touch. Hold for 15 seconds and repeat the stretch three times slowly.

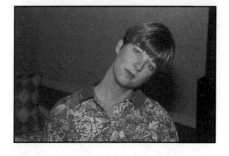

Head Rotation

This is the final stretch for our neck minders. Do the stretch slowly and smoothly, feeling the neck muscles stretch as you do it.

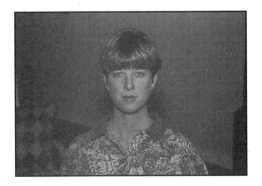

Photo 6-35. Relax, keeping your head pointed straight ahead.

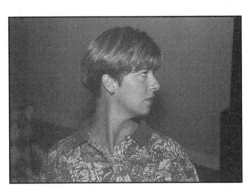

Photo 6-36. Take a deep breath, relax, and slowly turn your head to the side as far as it comfortably will go, feeling it stretch. Hold for 15 seconds.

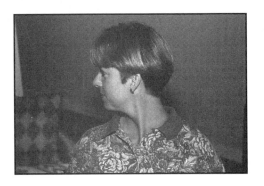

Photo 6-37. Take another deep breath, relax, and slowly turn your head so it's facing the other shoulder, as far as you can comfortably go. Hold for 15 seconds and repeat three times.

The Least You Need to Know

➤ Healthy stretching provides a mid-afternoon energy boost. As you stretch stiffness away, your muscles are also being nourished.

➤ Healthy stretching gives you a bridge of energy over the mid-afternoon blahs.

➤ Healthy stretching can be done anywhere and at any time.

➤ Pay attention to the signals your body is sending. Healthy stretching should be done before tension creeps in.

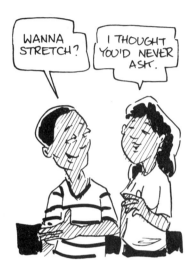

Chapter 7

Nightcaps:
To Be Shared
With Another

In This Chapter

➤ Two can be better than one—stretching with another

➤ Helping someone else helps yourself

➤ Healthy stretching for a good night's sleep

Two major points of this book are that healthy stretching doesn't have to be time-consuming and you don't need to buy expensive equipment. Healthy stretching blends into your normal daily endeavors and, so far, we've used doors, doorknobs, chairs, tables, and walls as stretching equipment.

This chapter is about healthy stretches you can enjoy as the day draws to a close. You will, however, need one piece of equipment for these stretches—but you may already have it on hand or can borrow one for awhile. It's a complex piece of equipment, usually weighing over 100 pounds, and perfect for the stretches I'll be showing you.

It goes by various names—husband, wife, significant other, life companion, or friend. With the built-in benefits of understanding your needs and the power to communicate, it's the ideal piece of equipment for healthy stretching.

Here are some things for you to consider about doing healthy stretching at night and with a partner:

➤ Stretching after a big dinner is usually not the ideal time.

➤ Choosing the right time depends on whether stretching stimulates or relaxes you. If it stimulates you, stretch earlier in the evening.

➤ The key is to find the best time for both stretching partners. One hour before bed usually works well.

➤ Communication is important, as one partner tells the other how far to go in the various stretch movements.

➤ The Nightcap stretches are gentle, yet you feel the results from head to toe.

➤ Mutual satisfaction is the result because each healthy stretch alternates between partners.

Chris's Concerns
The key to tandem stretches is communication and trust between partners. Do each stretch slowly, communicating with your partner on how far to stretch and when to stop. Stretch your partner only as far as he or she wants you to. Stretch, don't pull.

Back to Backs

It's time to reward your backs for the excellent service they performed all day, while at the same time conditioning them for a good night's sleep. If you think these are too strenuous for you, try the Hip Huggers group later in this chapter instead.

Extended Back Stretcher

This is a great healthy stretch to begin with, as it really feels very good. I would like to see both of you *alternate this stretch*: One supports while the other is stretched, and then reverse roles. Each partner should be stretched two times, holding for 15 seconds. Okay, I know it feels good, you can do this stretch three times if you prefer.

Begin by standing back to back with your heels about six inches apart from each other. Put your hands above your head and clasp them together.

To stretch Lisa, I lean slowly and gently forward, but only as far as she wants me to go. Lisa is on her toes and should not leave the ground. Along with the stretch in her back, she's also feeling the stretch in her abdominal area and oblique muscles. She's totally relaxed, allowing me to stretch her. Then I get to relax as we slowly change positions. Lisa slowly stretches me as she bends forward.

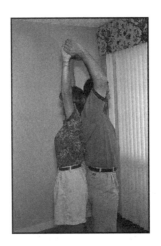

Photo 7-1. Because I'm taller then Lisa, it's okay for my arms to be bent.

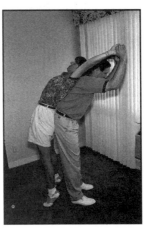

Photo 7-2. Lisa is totally relaxed, allowing me to stretch her out.

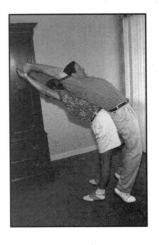

Photo 7-3. Notice how Lisa is extending her arms to pull me back.

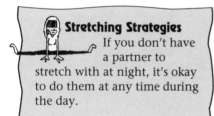

Stretching Strategies
If you don't have a partner to stretch with at night, it's okay to do them at any time during the day.

Extended Side to Side

Let's stretch from side to side and really feel it. This healthy stretch helps both partners at the same time. Follow the photos and stretch to each side, holding for 15 seconds in each stretched position. As you both stretch from side to side, you'll feel really good. Doing this stretch slowly and communicating with each other will help you both get maximum benefit from this wonderful stretch.

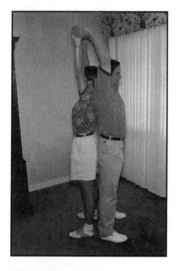

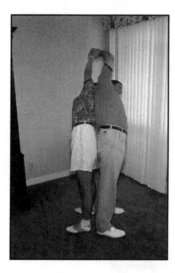

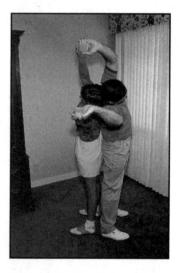

Photo 7-4. Begin by standing in the same position as Photo 7-1.

Photo 7-5. You can relax as the combined effort stretches both of you at the same time.

Photo 7-6. Slowly come back to the starting position and stretch the other side.

Suite Treats

The last two healthy stretches were done while standing, so now we'll sit down and do some rotational body stretches. You do remember that your body moves rotationally?

If you and your partner are mad at each other for any reason, you may want to skip these. It's not a time for an angry, "I'll get even with you" mentality. It's time for relaxation.

Back Rockers

Your lower back is going to feel so good after this. Remember to communicate and stretch slowly to get maximum benefit. Stretch, don't pull. Alternate the stretch for each partner holding 15 seconds with two or three repetitions. Stretching together is relaxing and fun—but please remember to communicate.

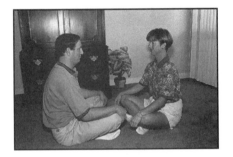

Photo 7-7. Start by sitting face to face, looking into your partner's eyes. Your feet are crossed in the campfire position.

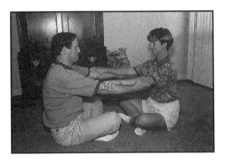

Photo 7-8. Extend your arms and grasp your partner's extended arms. Adjust for the size difference by grasping further up the arm, if needed.

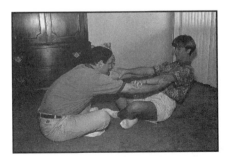

Photo 7-9. As Lisa slowly leans back, she's helping me stretch out my hips, lower back, and shoulders. I've communicated to her how I'm feeling and she's stretched me only as far as I want her to.

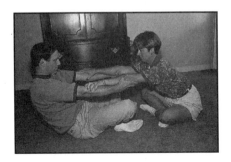

Photo 7-10. Slowly and gently we've changed positions. Lisa is now relaxed and stretching as I lean back only as far as she wants me to.

Seated Shoulder Stretchers

While in the same sitting position, you can now rotationally stretch the shoulders. Hold for 15 seconds and stretch only as far as comfortable. Please repeat two or three times.

Photo 7-11. Begin by sitting face to face, arms grasping each other as in Photo 7-8.

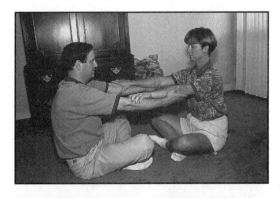

Photo 7-12. Lisa has rotated her left shoulder back, stretching my right shoulder forward.

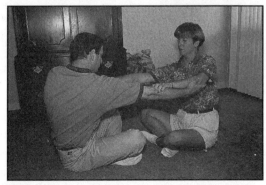

Photo 7-13. Slowly and gently we reverse as I rotate my right shoulder back. Lisa feels her left shoulder stretching forward.

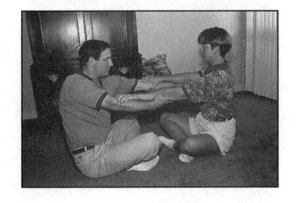

Togetherness Side-to-Side Stretches

Stay in the same seated position, but now stretch from side to side. Hold each stretched position 15 seconds, then stretch to the other side. Repeat this stretch two or three times.

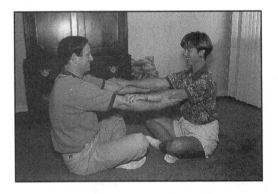

Photo 7-14. This stretch begins in cross-legged, arms-clasped position.

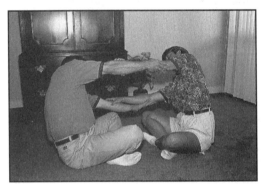

Photo 7-15. Gently and slowly, keeping your arms parallel, stretch to one side. Can you feel the stretch in your oblique muscles? Stretch only to the point where your partner wants to hold that position.

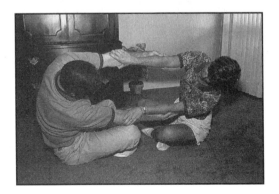

Photo 7-16. Now, slowly and gently stretch to the other side.

One-Arm Twist

As the last Suite Treat healthy stretch, let's do one more rotational stretch for our shoulders. Alternate positions holding for 15 seconds and repeat two or three times. Begin in the same cross-legged seated position but this time, hold only one arm as in Photo 7-17.

Photo 7-17. Lisa is holding my right arm as I hold her right arm. Because we are seated facing each other, they are on opposite sides.

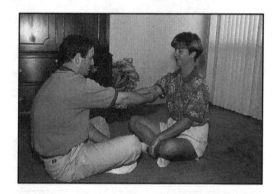

Follow the sequence in the next three photos for the One-Arm Twist.

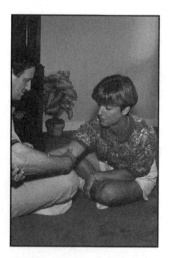

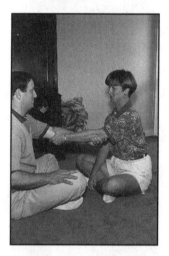

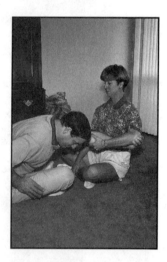

Photo 7-18. See how I've stretched Lisa's right shoulder by stretching her forward so her right shoulder almost touches my right knee. Without changing arms, we would now reverse so Lisa can help me stretch my right shoulder as she brings it toward her right knee.

Photo 7-19. Change arms so that each of you is holding the other's left arm.

Photo 7-20. Just as we did with the other arm, stretch each other's shoulder forward but, this time, to each other's left knee. You also may feel a stretch in your lower back.

Hip Huggers

While the following stretches are similar to the standing Back to Back stretches, it's a good idea to also do this series of healthy stretches. They feel so good and really continue the process of stretching out the large muscles of your back and upper body. And if you found that standing up and doing the Back to Back stretches were too strenuous for both of you, the Hip Huggers series can be done while seated.

Seated Back Stretchers

This series of healthy stretches will make you feel nice and relaxed while really providing your back, stomach, and abdomen with an easy-to-do stretch. Alternate stretches for each partner, holding 15 seconds and doing the stretch two or three times.

Begin by sitting back to back with your knees bent. Interlock your elbows together.

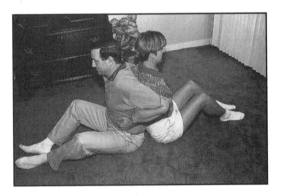

Photo 7-21. This is the position you should be in. Backs are touching and you're ready to stretch.

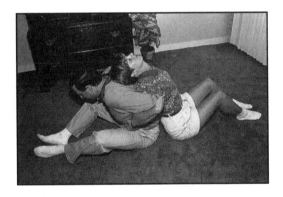

Photo 7-22. As I lean forward, Lisa is being stretched. Notice how her back is arched from her hips as she relaxes against my back.

Take turns stretching each other's back. Be sure to communicate with each other so that your partner stretches you only to a comfortable point.

Sitting Twist

Having fun so far? I thought so. Let's continue with a rotational twisting healthy stretch. Stretch each position for 15 seconds and alternate sides. Repeat two or three times.

Begin this stretch in the same back to back interlocking elbow position as shown in Photo 7-21.

Photo 7-23. We've both rotated to our left and feel the stretch in our oblique, torso, and back muscles. Now stretch to the other side.

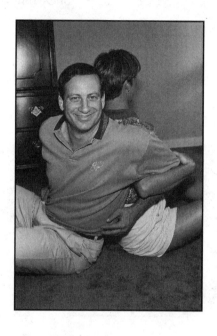

Chris's Concerns
As with all stretches done together, please communicate with each other. Please stretch your partner only as far as he or she wants you to.

Two for One

Partners can help each other with this group of healthy stretches for the main muscles of the legs. I think it's really important to have someone help you with this series. Each partner should be feeling wonderful by now because of the healthy stretches you've done so far. This group will stretch all the muscles affecting the hip.

Nighttime Knee Bender

Here's an easy one to begin with. Have your partner hold each position for 15 seconds. Alternate legs and repeat two or three times. Then you can switch positions. As with all stretches done together, please communicate with each other, and stretch your partner only as far as requested.

The partner being stretched first lies down on his or her back with one leg bent, foot on the floor. Grasp the knee and ankle of the other leg.

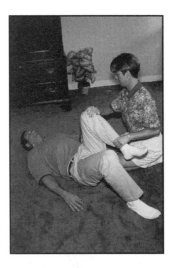

Photo 7-24. Lisa has grabbed the knee and ankle of my right leg. Also notice she has positioned herself on the side she will stretch.

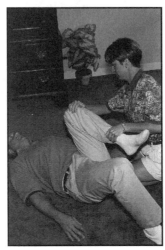

Photo 7-25. Lisa is now bringing my leg up toward my body, stretching the muscles of the hip.

Leg-Lifter, Two-Step Stretch

I dare you to say that ten times quickly out loud. But it is a good way to describe the benefits of this healthy stretch for your hamstrings. Alternate between each leg, holding the stretch positions for 15 seconds, and repeat two or three times. Then change places with your partner.

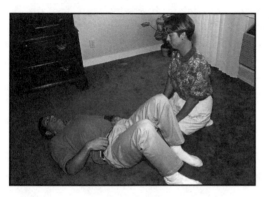

Photo 7-26. Begin by laying flat on the floor, both knees bent, and your partner on the side to be stretched first.

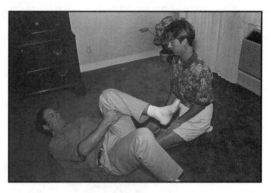

Photo 7-27. Reach with both hands and grab behind the knee.

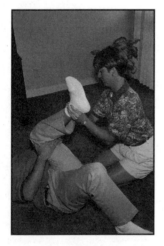

Photo 7-28. Stretch your leg up by pulling it back with your hands. Hold for a few seconds. Your partner can now hold your leg at the ankle and knee.

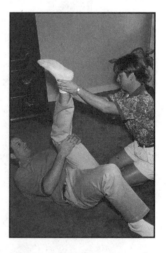

Photo 7-29. Slowly and gently, your partner pushes your ankle up, stretching your leg toward your chest.

Communicate to your partner what you're feeling. Ask your partner to move your leg to a position where you feel the stretching and not beyond.

Side Quad Stretch

This very effective quadriceps muscle healthy stretch helps lots of different problems related to discomfort in your lower body, back, and abdomen. The *quadriceps muscle* is the big muscle in the front of your thigh. A tight quadriceps muscle is a problem that affects most people's flexibility. Partners can really help each other with this stretch. Hold the stretch position 15 seconds, alternate legs, and repeat two or three times. Then switch positions. *To get the most benefit from the Side Quad stretch, don't arch your back as your partner pushes your knee back.*

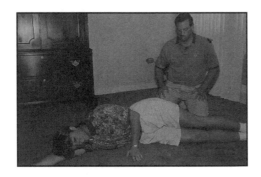

Photo 7-30. Lisa is laying on her side and I'm kneeling behind her.

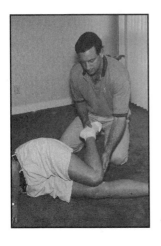

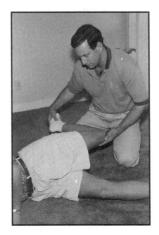

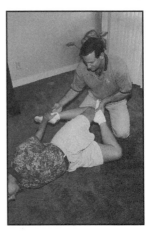

Photo 7-31. As Lisa bends her top leg back at the knee, I'm grasping the knee and ankle.

Photo 7-32. To stretch Lisa's quadriceps muscle, I'm slowly pulling her knee back and pushing her ankle toward her derrière. Lisa's ankle doesn't have to touch, just stretch toward her derrière. She's communicating how far to go.

Photo 7-33. Your partner should place the foot of the unstretched leg on the knee of the stretched one. Lisa is completing the stretch by reaching her top arm back, grasping her ankle, stretching as far as she wants. Hold for 15 seconds.

103

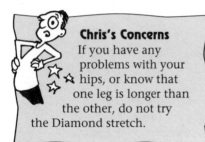

Chris's Concerns
If you have any problems with your hips, or know that one leg is longer than the other, do not try the Diamond stretch.

Diamond Stretch

Give your inner thighs and lower backs a diamond as you stretch them together with your partner. Hold each stretched position for 15 seconds.

Photo 7-34. Begin by sitting facing each other with your feet spread out and touching. Reach out and grab each other's hands keeping your back straight.

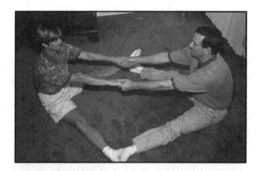

Photo 7-35. As Lisa leans back, she's pulling me forward, stretching out my lower back and inner thigh. My flexibility allows me to comfortably stretch farther than Lisa can.

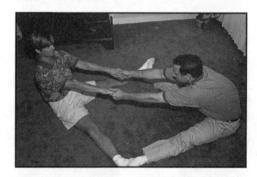

Photo 7-36. This is not a contest to see who can stretch farther. Each partner has the responsibility of following the other's instructions so each can benefit from the healthy stretches. Lisa is feeling the benefits of the stretch and has asked me to stop in this position.

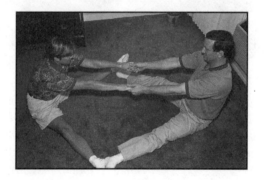

Last-Call Stretches

I really suggest you do these to finish an evening of healthy stretching. They're a less intense version of stretches you've already done, but it's a wonderful way to make sure you've really stretched your back, shoulders, and abdomen. You should enjoy a great night's sleep.

Soothing Gentle Back Stretch

Gentle and slow is the way to do this healthy stretch. Take deep breaths as your partner does all the work. Be sure and communicate how far to stretch each other. Alternate and repeat this stretch two or three times, holding for 15 seconds.

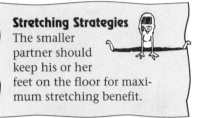

Stretching Strategies
The smaller partner should keep his or her feet on the floor for maximum stretching benefit.

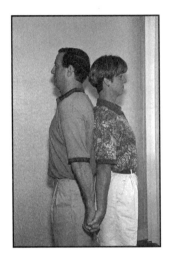

Photo 7-37. Begin by standing back to back, holding each other's hands at your sides.

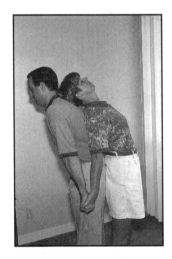

Photo 7-38. My gentle lean forward is stretching Lisa. Very gently is the key here.

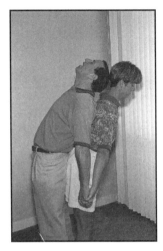

Photo 7-39. Now it's my turn. If you're the one being stretched, take deep breaths, relax, and enjoy.

Rotating Rhythm Stretch

You should be relaxing down now. Take deep breaths, join hands, and with a smile on both your faces, rotate through this healthy stretch. Hold each position for 15 seconds and slowly and rhythmically rotate as you stretch to the other side.

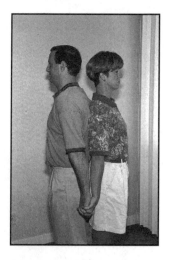

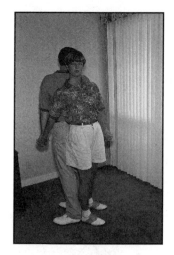

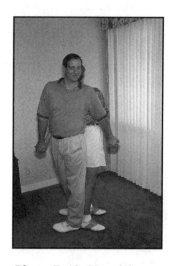

Photo 7-40. Begin by standing back to back, holding each other's hands at your side.

Photo 7-41. Slowly rotate to your right, keeping your feet and backs together. We were standing sideways but, as you can see, Lisa has now rotated and is facing you.

Photo 7-42. Now it's my turn to face you. I've rotated about 120 degrees, enjoying every degree. Take your time when you do any of the healthy stretches and enjoy them.

Curtain Call Stretch

You've done really well tonight, so I'll give you one last stretch. Take deep breaths and feel all the day's tension slip completely out of your system. Hold each stretch to the side for 15 seconds and repeat one or two times.

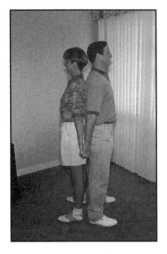

Photo 7-43. For the last healthy stretch of the night, stand back to back, holding hands at your sides.

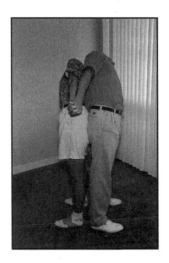

Photo 7-44. Keeping your shoulders and head together, slowly lean to one side. Take deep breaths as you hold for 15 seconds.

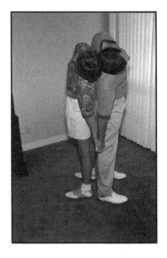

Photo 7-45. Slowly stretch to the other side. Take deep breaths and hold for 15 seconds.

The Least You Need to Know

➤ An hour before bedtime is a good time for the Nightcap stretches.

➤ Partners help each other stretch away the stress of the day.

➤ Healthy stretching partners must communicate and listen to their partner's instructions.

➤ Healthy stretching just before bedtime can help you have a wonderful night's sleep.

Part 3
Stretching for Real-Life Situations

The best way to stay flexible is to include healthy stretching in your day-to-day activities. It only takes a few minutes and I'll show you how to stretch right where you are.

If you're sitting in an office, involved in a physical profession, buckled into your airline seat, or waiting for your kids in the afternoon car pool, do something nice for yourself. I'm right here with you, so let's do them together.

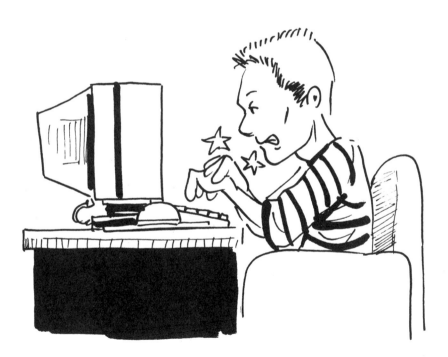

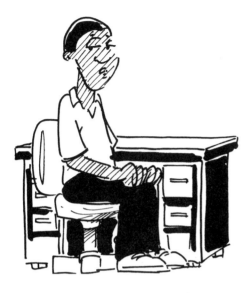

Chapter 8

Sitters of the World Unite! Get Vacationing Muscles Back to Work

In This Chapter

➤ I confess, Mr. Stretch, I'm a sitter

➤ It's not always the boss giving you that pain in the neck

➤ Stretching to prevent carpal tunnel syndrome

➤ Re-educate your sitting muscles

➤ Reboot your body

If you honestly analyze your day, you're probably surprised by the amount of time you spend sitting. Most people who have desk jobs realize they're chairbound. Some of you, however, believe your never-stop-for-a-minute day removes you from that category. "Mr. Stretch, I'm a busy person, do you think I just sit around all day with my feet up?" Actually, for some of you that would be an improvement. Putting your feet up occasionally can improve your circulation and flexibility.

You may be rushing from meeting to meeting, from power lunches to business dinners, but what do you do in meetings, at lunches, in your office, and while commuting. Sit! Unless you have an occupation that requires being on your feet, you're a "sitter." Your brain won't acknowledge it, but your muscles will. They've educated themselves to stay at the length best suited for accommodating your sitting needs. And when you can find time to participate in some physical activities, your muscles are not always ready to comfortably adapt to new requirements.

I suggest blending the healthy stretches in this chapter into your daily life. Since you hold a stretch for only 15 seconds, you probably can do most of them in a few minutes. You don't have to do them all at once either. We demonstrate the stretches in an office environment, proving how easily they fit into your real life.

These healthy stretches are designed to help specific problems sitters may experience. You may want to use them as preventative measures, helping to ward off tension headaches along with hip and back stiffness.

> **Stretching Strategies**
> As your personal stretching coach, I suggest keeping yourself full of energy with Chapter 6's Mid-Afternoon Energy Boosters.

It's Not Always the Boss Giving You That Pain in the Neck

> **Chris's Concerns**
> The Tension Deleter must be done slowly. When doing any neck stretches, it's very important to never jerk your neck. Stretching should be slow and deliberate.

Is there one person who doesn't rub their neck at least once a day to ease some sore stiff muscles? Maybe Gumby, but fictional characters don't count. Tension is a big reason we all get tight necks, but so is the fact that you're balancing a 12-pound object on your shoulders. Several muscle groups have the responsibility of allowing the head to move in various directions. We've already learned that as one group contracts, the other relaxes. And as the muscles work, they fatigue. Even normal use of our muscles requires healthy stretching.

Tension Deleter

The delete key on your computer keyboard gets rid of unwanted characters. This healthy stretch deletes neck tension. Stretch each side and hold for 15 seconds, repeating two or three times.

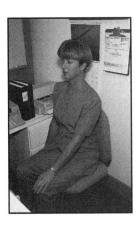

Photo 8-1. Sit up straight, back against the chair, hands on your knees. Concentrate on relaxing and take a few deep breaths.

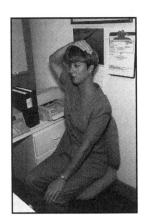

Photo 8-2. Place one hand on your head as Lisa is doing. The opposite hand resting on your knee determines how much stretch you'll get. If your neck is real tight, just keep your hand placed. If you're feeling loose but tension is creeping in, grasping the knee brings your shoulder down for increased stretching.

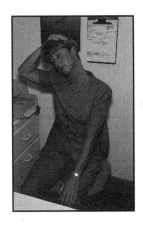

Photo 8-3. Pull your head in the direction of the pulling arm's shoulder. Lisa is using her right hand so she's feeling the stretch on her neck's left side down into the left shoulder.

One More Neck Stretch

This is such an easy stretch, it doesn't require a demonstration. You can do it when you're on the phone or sneak it in anytime the tension starts to mount.

Sit or stand up with good posture, head centered over your shoulders. Gently turn your head as far as you can to the left, hold for a few seconds, and slowly rotate it to the right. Repeat two or three times. Feel the muscles stretching and don't rush it.

Carpal Tunnel Syndrome: Curse of the Keyboard

Carpal tunnel syndrome is categorized by the World Health Organization as "a work-related musculoskeletal disorder." It's a painful disorder characterized by numbness, tingling, and pain in the base of the thumb and first three fingers, and is caused by constantly repeating movements of the wrists, hands, and fingers. Individuals who type on computer keyboards are in the high-risk category. Carpal tunnel syndrome is responsible for up to 40 percent of workers' compensation claims in the 1990s.

Computers are becoming a way of life and some of us spend hours typing away on our keyboards. Typing correspondence or business presentations are obvious examples of repetitive typing motions. Being on the Internet may be less obvious but is still a factor. It takes keystrokes to gain access to the wealth of information, and chat rooms are pure typing situations.

Your Mouse Gets Better Care Than You Do

Your mouse has a pad to cruise around on. By the way, using your mouse is also a cause of carpal tunnel syndrome: Your wrist and finger positions are repetitive and frequent. The best way to combat the syndrome is to prevent it. Try these suggestions:

➤ Purchase a pad your wrists can rest on while using the keyboard. They're available at computer and office supply stores.

➤ Replace your keyboard with a new ergonomic one designed to prevent the syndrome. *Ergonomic* is a technical term referring to the need and how the product was designed.

➤ You may want to purchase an ergonomic mouse to help prevent the syndrome.

➤ Take frequent rest periods if your hands are involved in any repetitive tasks.

➤ Do the healthy stretching exercises I've included to help prevent the syndrome.

Backhand Push

This first stretch is a simple one that you should do frequently throughout the day. Hold the position in Photo 8-5 for 15 seconds. Repeat this stretch two or three times whenever you're using your keyboard.

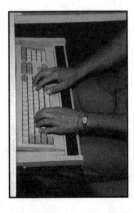

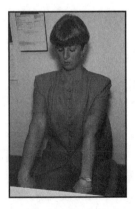

Photo 8-4. Even though this keyboard has a built-in wrist pad, the constant wrist angle and finger movements can cause problems.

Photo 8-5. Place the back of your hands against the edge of your desk. Straighten your arms and push forward until you feel the stretch on the back of your hands and the top of your wrist. This is the opposite position your hands are in when typing.

Wrist Relievers

To eliminate wrist muscle fatigue, a cause of carpal tunnel syndrome, do this healthy stretch during your keyboard rest periods. Hold each stretch for 15 seconds, repeating two or three times.

A word of warning: If you feel any sharp pain while doing these stretches, you may be experiencing the start of carpal tunnel syndrome. Please have your physician evaluate this situation. Therapy, which includes stretching, is readily available.

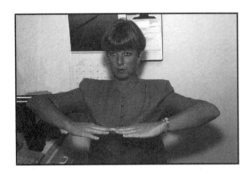

Photo 8-6. Begin with your arms in front, fingertips pointing at each other.

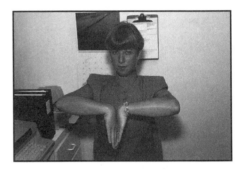

Photo 8-7. Slowly bring the backs of your hands together by rolling your fingers down until the wrists come together. Raise your hands slightly. The stretch should be felt from the fingers to the wrist.

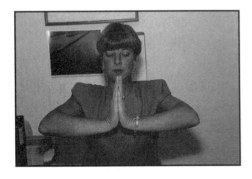

Photo 8-8. This stretch begins with your fingertips pointed to each other, arms at shoulder height, just like the last stretch. This time, however, slowly put pressure on the fingers, bringing your palms together.

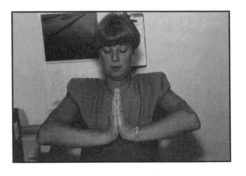

Photo 8-9. To balance your wrist muscles, the bottom of your wrists will feel this stretch as you lower your palms downward.

115

Re-Educating Your Sitting Muscles

As a "sitter," you've probably noticed that you get stiff at times. Sitting for long periods affects blood circulation. Blood tends to pool or accumulate in your lower extremities, like your feet. I wasn't joking before when I mentioned that some people might be better off if they could put their feet up now and then.

Sooner or later you have to do some walking and, as you recall, walking requires a rotational movement of your hip joints. These healthy stretches will also help your circulation, so let's make sure you keep the muscles in this area of your body flexible and ready.

> **Stretching Strategies**
> Should the Sitting Hip stretch cause a pulling in your inner thigh, consult Chapter 20, because your thighs are tighter or less flexible than your hips.

Sitting Hip Stretch

All you need is a chair for this stretch. If the Chapter 1 self-test indicated that you tend to walk with your feet pointed out like a waddling duck, this healthy stretch is one of the ways to correct that. Hold for 15 seconds, alternating crossed legs. Repeat two or three times.

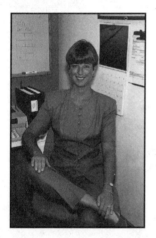

Photo 8-10. Begin by placing your right foot on your left leg. Rest your ankle on your thigh and put your right hand on your right knee.

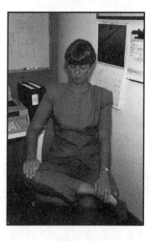

Photo 8-11. Push down on your right knee as you feel the hip muscle stretching. As flexibility increases, you'll notice your knee is lower when you cross your leg.

Sitting Outside Hip Stretch

Now let's do some stretching of the outside of your thigh, allowing you to rotate your upper body while you're rotating on your hip joint. Hold for 15 seconds and then stretch the other hip. I'd like to see you do this healthy stretch three times.

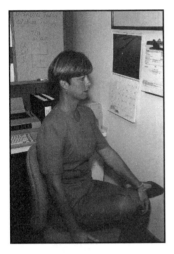

Photo 8-12. Place your right leg over your left to begin. Let your right hand relax by your side, left hand on leg.

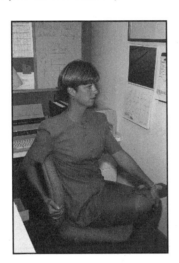

Photo 8-13. Put your right hand behind the chair and start to turn your upper body to the right. You'll feel this stretch in the front of your thigh, top of your hip, and lower back.

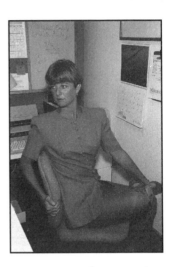

Photo 8-14. Continue the turn using your hands as leverage to feel the stretch. Only go as far as you can in order to hold the stretch for 15 seconds.

You Heard What?

If you've heard that early morning is a good time to try on a pair of shoes you want to buy, that is wrong. People tend to either sit or stand most of the day causing some blood to remain in their lower extremities, swelling their feet and ankles. It may not be a lot, but it's there. Comfortably fitting shoes in the morning become just the opposite in the afternoon. For a more comfortable fit overall, buy new shoes in the afternoon.

Quad Muscle Wake-Up

Quadricep muscles will adapt to your sitting for long periods of time and will shorten. You need to stretch and re-educate them to maintain a longer length. This is the number one area where almost everyone is less flexible. Hold the stretch for 15 seconds and then change sides. Repeat two times.

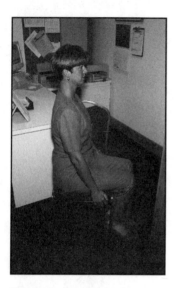 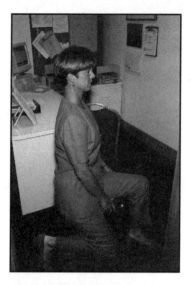 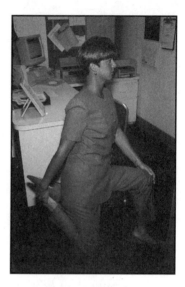

Photo 8-15. Begin by sitting in your chair. You will need to use one that will allow you to sit half on, half off. Or, sit sideways as Lisa is doing.

Photo 8-16. Adjust to the position where you have one leg on the chair while you rest the other knee on the floor.

Photo 8-17. Reach down and grasp your ankle, pulling it back so you could draw a straight line through your shoulder, hip, and knee.

Leg Stretch

Your legs are attached to your hips, so let's take a minute or two to work on their flexibility. *If you sit all day, both your hamstrings and hip flexor muscle groups will shorten.* You haven't shortened the muscles by fatiguing them as a result of use; instead, long periods of time spent sitting have programmed their shortness. This requires re-education by healthy stretching.

Do this next stretch slowly, hold for 15 seconds, and repeat for the other side. Be sure to choose a chair that won't move when you put your foot up. Select one that will allow your foot to stay below your hips.

Chris's Concerns
When doing these standing hamstring stretches slowly, stop immediately if you feel pressure in your lower back. It may pinpoint a problem you're not aware of in your back that your doctor should evaluate.

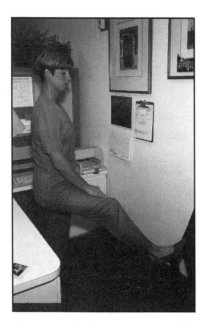

Photo 8-18. *You need to stand up to stretch the hamstrings. Put your foot on a chair that can't move easily and extend your leg to a slightly bent position.*

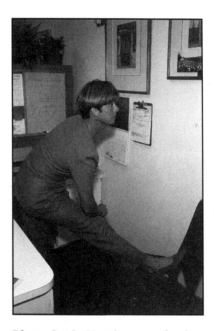

Photo 8-19. *Keeping your back straight, lean forward toward your knee. Lisa has her elbow on her leg to prevent her from stretching too far. You will feel the stretch on the back of your thigh up through your derrière.*

Hamstring Standing Stretch

One more time for those hamstrings. Hold this stretch for 15 seconds, alternating legs. I'd like to see you stretch on each side three times.

Photo 8-20. Stand straight with one foot out in front with the toe raised up to where it's comfortable.

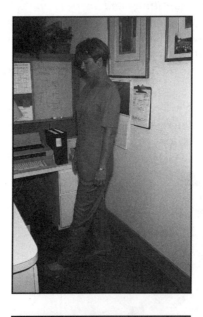

Photo 8-21. Put your hands on your knee and slowly lean forward, feeling the stretch in the back of your thigh.

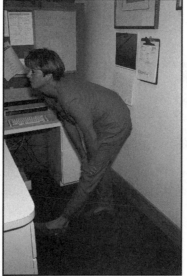

Reboot Your Body

Your upper body can use a little reprogramming as a result of sitting. I assume you have a computer you can use (for holding-onto purposes only, so don't run out and buy one). If not, find something to hold onto that's about the same height as a monitor.

Programmer Stretch 1

I'm assuming you're in front of your computer monitor when you plan on doing this healthy stretch. By the way, where did you get that screen saver? You will enjoy this stretch as it loosens up your shoulder and upper back muscles. Hold for 15 seconds and repeat as many times as you wish.

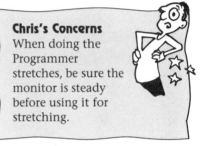

Chris's Concerns
When doing the Programmer stretches, be sure the monitor is steady before using it for stretching.

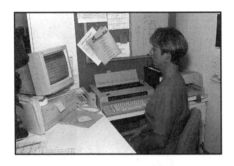

Photo 8-22. Begin by sitting straight facing your monitor.

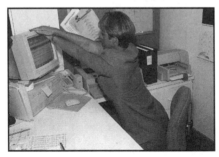

Photo 8-23. Cross your hands and extend your arms while holding gently on to the top of the monitor.

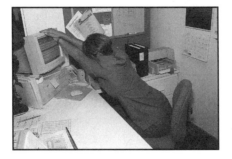

Photo 8-24. Lean forward until you can feel the stretching in your back muscles.

Programmer Stretch 2

This healthy stretch will help your flexibility as it reboots your upper body. Begin as you did in Photo 8-22, by facing your monitor and sitting up straight. Take a few deep breaths to relax. Alternate each side, holding for 15 seconds, and repeat for a total of two or three times.

Photo 8-25. Place one hand on top of the monitor.

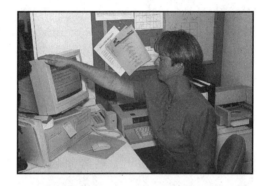

Photo 8-26. Keeping your head facing the screen, and your feet on the floor to prevent the chair from swiveling, raise your other hand and slowly rotate it back until you feel some pressure. Hold for 15 seconds. Only go as far back as comfortable.

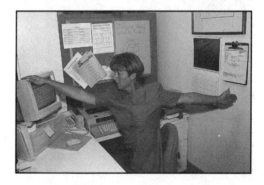

The Least You Need to Know

➤ Sitting for long periods of time can adversely affect your flexibility.

➤ Neck tightness can occur just from supporting and balancing your head.

➤ Carpal tunnel syndrome is responsible for up to 40 percent of workers' compensation claims.

➤ Healthy stretching and using a wrist pad can help protect you.

➤ Lower body muscles will reprogram themselves to stay short if you don't re-educate them with healthy stretching.

➤ Healthy stretching will keep your muscles flexible and alert, ready to move.

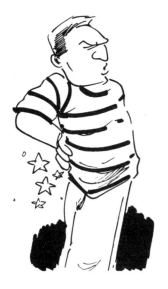

Chapter 9

Physical Professions or Hobbies: Stiffness, Stiffness Everywhere

In This Chapter

➤ Healthy stretching for physical labor

➤ Athletes have it easy, compared to you

➤ Saving your knees, backs, and arms

➤ Mr. Stretch works with the weekend gardener

➤ Eliminating backaches caused by physical labor

Okay, sports fans, we're in the closing seconds of the Super Bowl. Fred, the carpenter, takes the snap from Joan, the weekend gardener. He fakes a handoff to Sybil, the painter, and throws downfield to Barry, the telephone lineman, who climbs over Otis, the mason, to make the winning catch.

What I'm trying to illustrate is that when you physically use your body for work or hobbies, it's similar to how athletes use theirs. Athletes are put on the "Physically unable to perform disabled list" when they pull muscles or suffer injuries. In some sports, baseball for example, practice is limited to only an hour or two a day plus the game. I assume you work a lot longer than that.

Compared to You, Million-Dollar Athletes Have it Easy

Now let's talk about you. You may be putting more stress on your body than athletes do, since you're doing multiple kinds of tasks as well as repetitive work. An athlete tends to be more specialized by choice of sport. A carpenter, on the other hand, has to lift and carry heavy objects and bend, stoop, or climb to fasten them in place. Unless the carpenter's using a nail gun, arm bending comes into play as the hammer pounds the nails.

Mr. Stretch Explains

Arthritis is defined as an inflammation of the joints. It can be caused by infection, or be *metabolic* (meaning the effect of years and years of use), or the result of how your bones interact. If you're suffering serious pain or if arthritis runs in your family, I strongly suggest you consult your doctor.

Stretching Strategies

While it's important to do the healthy stretches before starting any physical labor, it's extremely important to also do some of them after you're done. Muscles become fatigued with use and shorten. Healthy stretching, after working, returns muscle groups to their proper length reducing or eliminating the soreness you would probably feel the next day.

As athletes have developed their bodies, based on their specific sport, you have too. Repetitive motions like painting, hammering, or laying tile use one side of your body. If you're working with only your right side, what happens to your left? It's unbalanced.

To compound the problem, chances are you've done the same things for many years. I find many athletes develop problems later in their careers. (In most sports, late 20s is getting old.) How about a 35-year-old carpenter or a 42-year-old weekend gardener? You've had a longer time to develop hidden problems. Only they aren't hidden forever, as those increasing aches and pains demonstrate. It's easy to blame some of the aches on *arthritis* or some other medical reason. However, some aches and pains can be attributed to lack of flexibility and muscle imbalance.

Athletes are raising their performance levels and extending their careers simply because many are including flexibility training earlier in life as part of their conditioning programs. Why should you be any different? You may see lots of healthy stretches demonstrated in this chapter and feel you don't have time to do them. Here's why you'll want to:

➤ Keep in mind that the holding position is only 15 seconds.

➤ In a few minutes, you can perform some preventive maintenance protecting your muscles and joints.

➤ You can sneak them in all day long.

➤ Healthy stretching feels good immediately.

I'll be demonstrating the healthy stretches in this chapter right on the job site, proving you can do healthy stretching in a real-life situation. These healthy stretches are especially important if you perform physical labor only on weekend projects, shovel snow occasionally, or work in your garden intermittently. Muscles require education to prepare for the work ahead. Believe me, it's far better to take a few minutes now than suffer later.

Lifters: Mr. Stretch Helps You Carry the Load

Having confidence in your body's ability to handle workload situations is extremely important. The healthy stretches I demonstrate are the same ones I've instituted with my corporate clients to help their workforce prepare for the day's activities. It's amazing how their workforce started becoming aware of their bodies. Healthy stretching before working helped prevent injuries. They also learned how stretching eliminated their aches and pains, preventing an escalation of a problem into a full-blown injury, thus lowering workers' compensation claims.

Lifters are especially vulnerable to injuries. You put lots of stress on your back, hips, and shoulders. These healthy stretches will help prevent injury as well as increase your energy levels.

Lower Body Standing Stretch

Lifting should be done with your legs, so let's begin with some healthy stretches for that area. This is an easy stretch to do on site—you can use a ladder, scaffolding, or even a pile of stacked material like lumber. Hold the stretched position for 15 seconds and alternately stretch each leg two times.

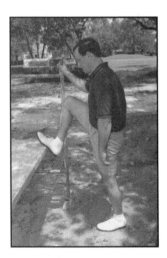

Photo 9-1. I'm using some scaffolding as I place one foot almost waist high on the surface, while still standing straight.

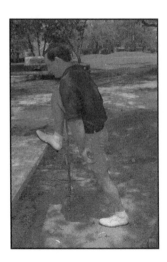

Photo 9-2. Lean into your front leg to feel the stretch in the hamstrings of the raised leg as well as the standing leg's quadricep muscle.

125

Hamstring Conditioner

As you do the Hamstring Conditioner, please do it slowly, feeling the hamstring of the raised leg gently stretch as you reach the 15 second hold position. Never jerk into any healthy stretch. One other suggestion, keep the raised leg slightly bent. It helps prevent unneeded stress on any unknown problems you may have with your lower back.

Hamstrings are usually left out while you're lifting. Their help is not usually required. But sometimes they are needed and this healthy stretch helps prevent the discomfort that could arise from tearing this huge muscle. Hold for 15 seconds and alternate legs to stretch both hamstrings two times.

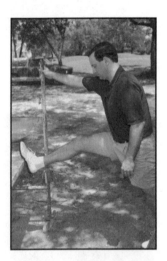

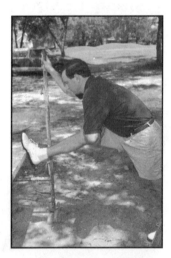

Photo 9-3. Place your foot on a higher surface (but below your waist), like scaffolding or a stack of materials. Notice that my raised leg is slightly bent.

Photo 9-4. Slowly lean into the raised leg lowering your body down as close to your leg as you can comfortably go. Keep your back straight and you'll feel the hamstring of the raised leg stretching.

Standing Quad Conditioner

You need your quadriceps, the big muscles in the front of your thigh, for lifting. This muscle group helps provide the leverage for lifting and is subject to injury. Please stretch both quadriceps muscles two times. Alternate legs and hold the stretch for 15 seconds.

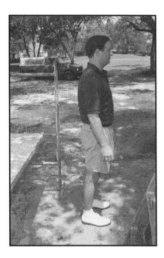

Photo 9-5. Stand more than an arm's length away from a raised surface, with your back to it. Raise your leg backward (not pictured), placing the top of your foot on the raised surface.

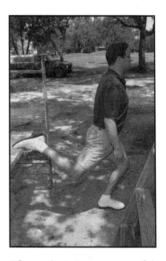

Photo 9-6. Lower your hips as you bend the standing leg, keeping erect so you don't lean forward. If you don't feel the stretch in the raised leg's quad muscle, stand farther away from the raised surface.

Inner-Thigh Conditioner

This is one muscle group that a lot of construction workers and weekenders seem to strain a lot. It's a nagging kind of injury that can put you in an irritable mood, affecting the quality of your work. Do it slowly, following the sequence of photos on the next page from Photo 9-7 to 9-11. Hold the stretched position for 15 seconds. Alternate the stretch for both legs two times.

Stretching Strategies

The torso stretching portion of the Quad Conditioner provides the opportunity to healthily stretch another group of muscles prone to injury for lifters. Your torso, or upper body, has to be flexible enough to participate in the lifting process. You can also do another stretch by slowly bending and reaching sideways behind the position of your raised leg.

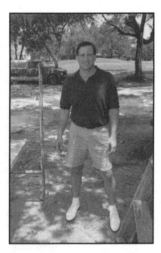

Photo 9-7. Stand sideways to the scaffolding or other raised surface.

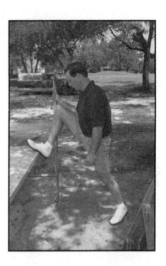

Photo 9-8. This time, as I put my foot on the raised surface, my standing foot remains sideways to it.

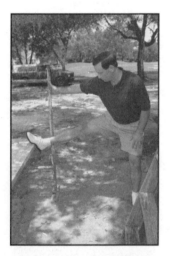

Photo 9-9. Adjust your body away from the surface so you can straighten the raised leg to a slightly bent position.

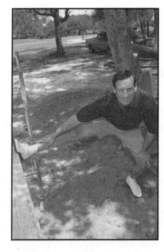

Photo 9-10. As you bend your standing leg down slowly, you'll feel the stretch in the inner thigh of the raised leg. Hold 15 seconds in this position.

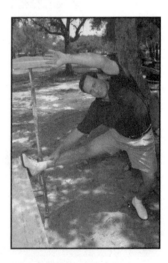

Photo 9-11. You can also do a torso stretch by leaning your shoulders slowly so you can reach and hold onto the raised ankle. Hold for 15 seconds.

Arm Benders: Join Mr. Stretch at the Bar

I'm going to treat you to a few healthy stretches—not drinks. By having to bend and rotate your arm repeatedly, you probably have *weak triceps* and *overused biceps*. This imbalance results in tightness in the front of the elbow where the biceps' tendon attaches and where it gets used a lot. The following healthy stretches will help you condition both muscle groups. If you use your arms a lot, I suggest also doing these stretches immediately after finishing your work, realigning both muscle groups to their proper lengths.

If you occasionally work on home projects requiring repeated arm movements, like painting the guest room or refinishing the dining room table, you really need to do these. I'm using a scaffolding bar but you can use a tightly secured towel bar or other horizontal object that you can wrap your hands around.

> **Mr. Stretch Explains**
> *Weak triceps* and *overused biceps* can be a result of using your arm repetitively. Triceps are the muscles in the back of your upper arm; biceps are the opposing muscles in the front of the arm. Both are connected to the elbow and shoulder.

One-Armer Stretch

This can be a two-step stretch depending on your flexibility. Sometimes just extending the arm out to the side and holding on to something as you move away stretches the biceps. I suggest holding for 15 seconds in both stretched positions to stretch the biceps and the shoulder. Alternate arms and stretch each arm two times.

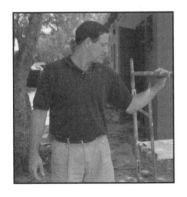

Photo 9-12. Stand sideways to the bar and grab it from underneath with one hand, keeping your elbow bent. Your head is turned toward the bar.

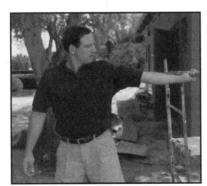

Photo 9-13. I straighten my arm as I slowly lean away from the bar, feeling the stretch in my biceps. Hold for 15 seconds.

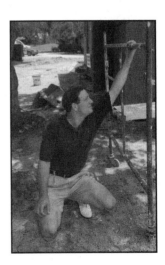

Photo 9-14. Slowly and gently lower yourself as you feel your shoulder muscles beginning to stretch

129

Double-Handed Stretch

This healthy stretch helps your arms where they attach to the torso. Please do this stretch slowly, feeling the stretching sensation increase all the way to your shoulders and chest. Hold for 15 seconds and stretch two times.

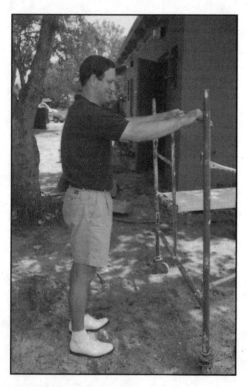

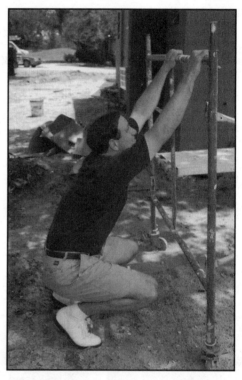

Photo 9-15. Stand facing the bar, gripping it with both hands from the top.

Photo 9-16. Slowly lower yourself to your knees, feeling the stretch all the way through your arms, armpits, and into your chest and upper back.

Backward Arm Conditioner

Arm benders tend to develop problems with *biceps tendonitis*, a swelling of the tendon where it attaches to the elbow, usually brought on by repetitive use. This healthy stretch is preventative as well as a conditioner for other muscle groups needed for arm bending and rotating. This time you'll need to hold a bar *vertically,* allowing your thumb to be on the bottom and your little finger on top. Hold the stretched position for 15 seconds. Alternate arms and stretch both two times.

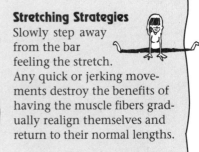

Stretching Strategies
Slowly step away from the bar feeling the stretch. Any quick or jerking movements destroy the benefits of having the muscle fibers gradually realign themselves and return to their normal lengths.

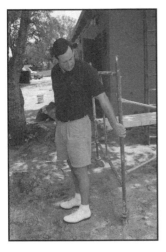

Photo 9-17. With your back to the bar, reach back and grab the outside of the bar with one hand, thumb down, little finger up.

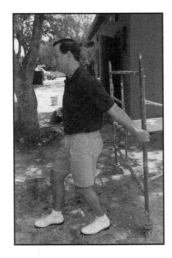

Photo 9-18. Step away from the bar slightly, straightening the arm.

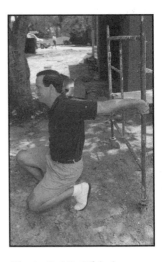

Photo 9-19. This is a continuation of the stretching position, if you are very flexible. If not, try to reach a position halfway between Photo 9-18 and Photo 9-19. Slowly drop to one knee, keeping your arm straight. You'll really feel this stretch through the middle of your biceps.

131

Mr. Stretch Explains
Overuse syndrome occurs when performing a repetitive activity for such a long period of time it creates an injury. It doesn't happen at any one time, you didn't feel a muscle pull or tear, and you didn't hear a "popping" sound. You realized something was wrong when you woke up the next morning and couldn't lift your arm because it was so sore.

Benders: Mr. Stretch Plants the Seeds for Healthy Stretching

If you enjoy gardening but not the sore muscles that can be a result, the stretches in this section might just prevent that pain in your back. You are every bit as much a Weekend Warrior as those who sit around most of the week and then physically exercise on the weekends. Maybe you even garden and physically exercise, a potential hybrid of double trouble.

Thinking more about the beautiful flowers and luscious vegetables that your garden will produce than what you're doing to your body is a sure-fire recipe for trouble. Just as you want to keep pests out of your garden, I want to keep some other pests out of your body—like strained muscles, wrenched backs, and sore hips. You'll remember the growing season for giant tomatoes, not giant backaches.

You Heard What?

If you hear people say they don't risk injury doing a few things in the garden, they're wrong. Anyone who does a little activity for an extended period of time may not realize it, but it becomes a big activity for your body. It's amazing how much time it takes to do even just a few simple gardening tasks, besides consider the positions you're asking your body to hold. Stooping and bending over are not normal positions. Hoeing, shoveling, or raking may make you think you're feeling good doing some work, but your body's not ready for it. We know muscles have to adapt to accommodate your needs, but how quickly can they change? Healthy stretching educates them to be ready, willing and able to help.

Back Planter

Being on your hands and knees and extending your back is not the normal comfort range for your muscles. This healthy stretch extends your back while providing some muscle education to help keep you gardening without pain. It really helps avoid the *overuse syndrome*. Use a towel or pad for your knees. Uncomfortable knees will not allow you to concentrate on feeling the stretch. Repeat the stretch two times, holding the stretch positions for 15 seconds.

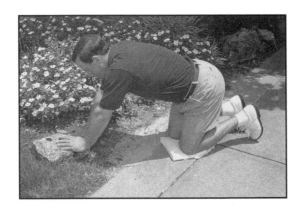

Photo 9-20. Get down on your hands and knees. Rest your hands on a rock or something you can hold in front of you.

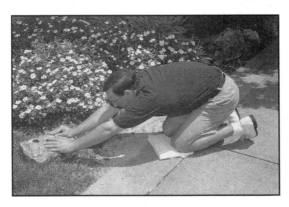

Photo 9-21. Stretch back, touching your derrière to your heels, and feeling the stretch starting in your upper body. Hold for 15 seconds.

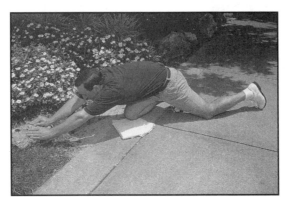

Photo 9-22. Alternate taking each leg back holding for 15 seconds.

Both Sides Body Conditioner

If you use only one side of your body, it tends to get tighter because you've overused it. This healthy rotational stretch equalizes both sides. Hold for 15 seconds and stretch each side two or three times.

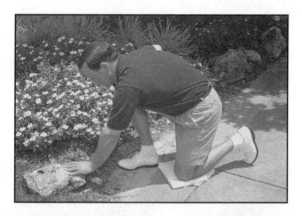

Photo 9-23. Place one knee on the ground with the hand on the same side holding on to something in front of you. The other knee should be bent with the foot farther forward.

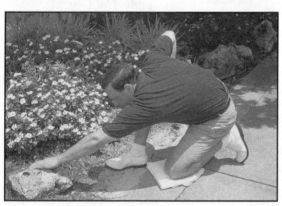

Photo 9-24. Place your opposite hand on your knee and lean back on your heels. You'll feel your shoulders rotate and stretch as you go back.

Hamstring Planter

When you're bending, hamstrings—the big muscles in the back of your thigh—need to be flexible, allowing your hips to move. If your hips can't easily move, it usually causes back pressure and you know what that means—backaches! Hold the stretch position for 15 seconds. Switch legs and repeat for a total of two times for each side. Let Mr. Stretch show you how backaches can be a thing of the past!

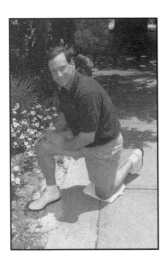

Photo 9-25. Begin by putting one knee on the ground and bending the other knee with the foot farther forward.

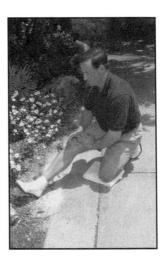

Photo 9-26. Move your foot forward so it's straight out with your knee slightly bent.

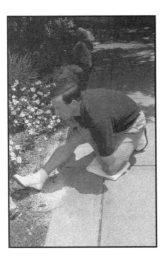

Photo 9-27. Lean forward slowly feeling the hamstring stretch. Only stretch as far as you feel comfortable, holding for 15 seconds.

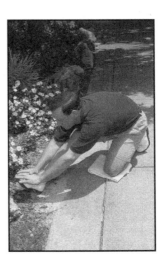

Photo 9-28. Reach your hands out toward your ankles and stretch forward holding for 15 seconds.

135

Stop the Presses! Mr. Stretch Shows Backache to Be a Thing of the Past

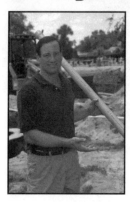

Photo 9-29. Chris "Mr. Stretch" Verna.

Dateline, Boca Raton, Florida: Chris "Mr. Stretch" Verna today shocked the world by announcing that backaches due to muscle strains from physical work can be eliminated. Reporters were stunned when he demonstrated some healthy stretching using PVC plumbing pipe on his shoulders and were further taken aback when he added: "It works just as well with a rake, broom, hoe, or baseball bat." The assembled media knowingly nodded to each other, though, as he also revealed the catch associated with their use—injuries will occur to spectators standing within the turning radius of the pipe.

Pipe Bender Stretch

Hope you're having as much fun with this Guide as I am. I really think that lots of backaches and loss of work can be avoided by doing a few healthy stretches for your back. They're easy and you can use whatever is available for equipment. Building sites are laden with pieces of PVC pipe, electrical conduits, etc. Do I need to include the warning not to use them if they've already been installed? Also, I wasn't just kidding that people can be injured if they're standing in the radius of the pipe as you turn. So please go off by yourself to do these healthy stretches, just to be safe.

Please do them slowly, stopping at the stretch position for the count of two. Using pipe, a broom, or similar objects for the two pipe stretches increases the range of your turn. Not having something in your hands limits the rotation. I'd like you to repeat this exercise slowly about five times.

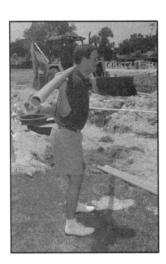

Photo 9-30. Hold the pipe in a balanced position on your shoulders.

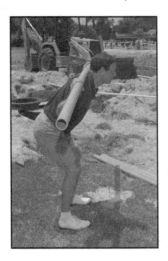

Photo 9-31. Start bending forward slowly, keeping your knees slightly bent.

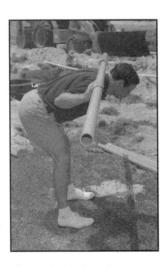

Photo 9-32. Bend way forward, keeping your back straight, so that your back is almost parallel to the ground. Hold for a count of two.

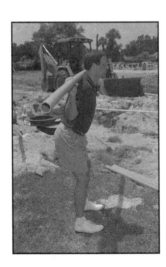

Photo 9-33. Stand back up.

Pipe Twister Stretch

Moving our bodies, as we have learned, is accomplished by rotating around our joints. This final healthy rotating stretch, combined with the previous one, will help prevent lower back strain while you work. Please do it slowly and concentrate on feeling the stretch working. Hold each stretched position for 15 seconds and then rotate to the stretched position for the other side. Repeat slowly three times.

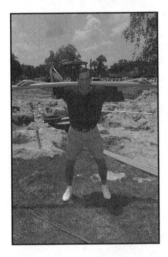

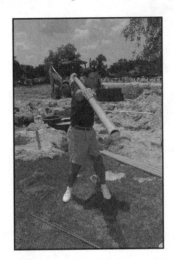

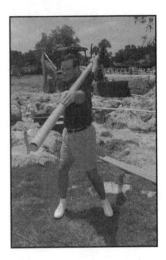

Photo 9-34. Stand up straight, knees slightly bent, hand wrapped over the top of the pipe. Extend your arms down the pipe as far as you can.

Photo 9-35. Rotate your body to one side so that one side of the pole faces to the front or beyond. Stretch—don't whirl it there.

Photo 9-36. Rotate to the other side slowly.

The Least You Need to Know

➤ Your body may experience more stress than a star athlete's does.

➤ On-the-job injuries can be reduced by healthy stretching.

➤ Healthy stretching can help prevent the overuse syndrome.

➤ Even simple activities like gardening require healthy stretching muscle re-education.

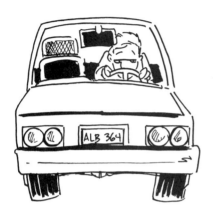

Chapter 10

Captured Commuters

In This Chapter

➤ Surviving air travel with mental and physical flexibility

➤ Staying alert in your car

Ode to the Captured Commuter

Behind the wheel, stuck in your seat,
Or are you trapped at 30,000 feet?
You may think you're going from here to there—
To your body, you're not going anywhere.
So as you travel far and wide
Your big muscles start to hide…
Getting tighter and shorter too.
Gee, I'm glad to be with you,
'Cause while you're sitting in that chair
And not really going anywhere…
Mr. Stretch will bring you a treat—
Some healthy stretching in your seat.

The 30,000-Feet Energy Secret

How do you feel when you leave the plane after a two-hour or longer trip? Lethargic, sleepy, stiff? You're probably thinking about a nice comfortable bed to drag yourself into.

But who are those other people getting off the same plane, looking so refreshed and perky, ready to close a big deal or spend a night on the town? Could that orange-bordered book sticking out of their carry-on bags be the secret to their energy? It's easy to find out, since you're reading it now.

Stretching, unlike other forms of exercise, can be done almost anywhere. While there is a time and place to do strength and aerobic exercises, healthy stretching keeps you alert and full of energy and easily blends into your lifestyle—even when confined to an airline seat. By doing a few healthy stretches en route, you help prevent your muscles from fatiguing and making you feel the same way.

A 45-Million-Dollar Stretching Machine

Yes, that's right, I'm going to demonstrate some healthy stretches you can do right in your seat or in the aisle. Don't worry about annoying your fellow passengers—after all, you're not exactly a screaming baby. Maybe some of them will want to join in. But if you're flying on business, don't share these stretches with your competitors.

Airline seats come in one-size-fits-all. That's why you get the feeling you're sliding out of your seat when the support's in the wrong location for your particular physique. A rounding of the *spine*, almost like a "C" shape, causes your *vertebrae* to put pressure on the *discs* and results in an uncomfortable pinching feeling.

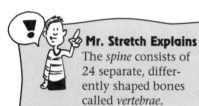

Mr. Stretch Explains
The *spine* consists of 24 separate, differently shaped bones called *vertebrae*. Between each pair of vertebrae is a *disc* of cartilage, a material that cushions the bones during movement. Serious back problems usually involve some damage or rupture of the disc material.

If you've ever fallen asleep on the plane, you'll wake up feeling a little stiffer than normal. It's not because you're just sitting and sleeping, it's because you're in the wrong position. It's even worse than being a "sitter." You can do a few things to help:

➤ Remove wallets or other items from back pockets that can produce discomfort by pressing against your muscles or making one side tilt, putting you out of muscle balance.

➤ Take your shoes off while flying.

➤ Wear loose comfortable clothing.

➤ Do some healthy stretching during the flight to keep your muscles from becoming fatigued.

➤ Drink water every hour during the flight.

Psychologically, you feel smaller on a plane because of the cramped conditions and unfamiliar people nearly on top of you. Even in an aisle seat where people keep passing you, you may develop a feeling of being crowded or becoming smaller. Flexibility makes you feel bigger and wider. So the healthy stretches are really important in order to maintain your mental as well as physical sense of flexibility.

The Fighter Pilot Stretch

Want to learn some stretches pilots are taught? Fluids pool in legs from the inactivity of sitting, a problem even combat pilots face. Since gravity makes fluids seek the lowest level, feet and ankles swell.

Pilots are taught to counteract gravity by pushing the fluids back up, not allowing it to pool in their feet. It begins by squeezing the muscles in your toes and arches by *contracting* (voluntarily tightening) them. This pushes the blood out of your feet. Then squeeze the calves by pointing the toes up and then down, along with your thigh muscles, to get the pooled blood back circulating. You may want to do the Fighter Pilot stretch a few times during the trip.

Flaps-Up Arm Stretch

Most of the time while you're sitting, your arms are by your sides, also collecting fluids. This stretch makes your whole body longer as you raise your arms above your head. Hold for 15 seconds and repeat two or three times.

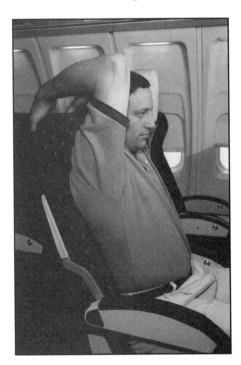

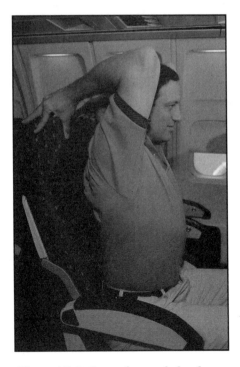

Photo 10-1. Sit up tall in your seat as you reach both arms back over your head. Hold onto your headrest. I'm already feeling the stretch in my arms and upper back.

Photo 10-2. Lean forward slowly, taking your back and shoulders off the seat. You'll feel the stretch in your chest, torso, arms, and shoulder blades.

141

Banking Rotation

This healthy stretch deals with the extended length of time your body stays in one position. The rotation in the stretch reminds the body that it must still be prepared for the rotation required in moving. Do each side two times, holding for 15 seconds. I'm demonstrating the stretch in an aisle seat but it can be done in any seat.

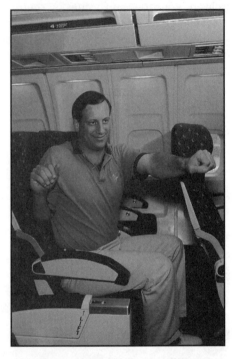

Photo 10-3. Put one arm straight out on the seat in front. Bend your other arm and position it slightly behind you on the seat-back for leverage.

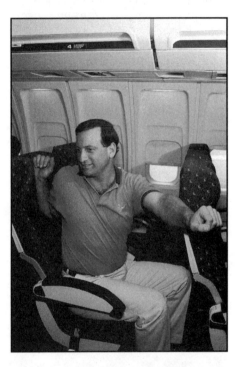

Photo 10-4. Rotate to the side so that your upper body turns and you feel the twisting stretch in your torso.

Landing Gear Neck Stretch

Necks seem to be the biggest problem I see with people flying. Because you're not sitting in the correct positions for long periods of time, your neck develops some problems. Use your legs, your landing gear, for leverage in this healthy stretch. Do each side three times, alternating between stretches and holding for 15 seconds. (If you're sitting in an emergency aisle, never use the emergency exit door or handle for leverage.)

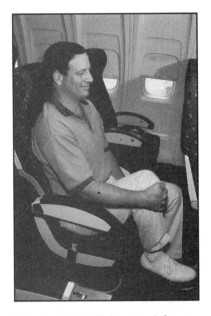

Photo 10-5. Sitting straight, grab one knee with the arm on the same side of the body.

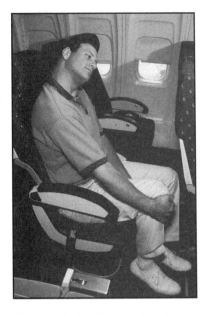

Photo 10-6. Tilt your head toward the opposite shoulder.

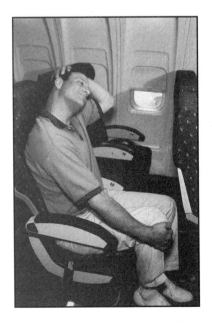

Photo 10-7. For more of a stretch, reach up, placing your free hand on the other side of your head. Slowly stretch, trying to bring your head closer to the shoulder. You'll feel this stretch from your ear to your shoulder.

Serving-Tray, Shoulder-Blade Stretch

As you sit, the muscles located between your shoulder blades get tight and tense. Stretch some of that tension away using the seat in front of you. Do this gently, not only for your sake, but also for the person occupying the seat. Stretch three times, holding for 15 seconds.

Photo 10-8. Criss-cross your extended arms and rest them on the serving tray in the up position on the seat in front of you. Push your shoulders forward and try to create a feeling of more space between your shoulder blades.

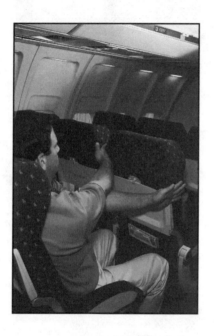

Mr. Stretch Explains
Even though you may think your spine is straight, it's not designed that way. Body support and the needs for rotational movements evolved it into a more functional "S" shape. Stand with your heels against a wall. You should feel a gap or arch right above your hips. Your shoulders should touch the wall, with another gap at your neck. In other words, an "S" shape.

Tail-Section Stretch

Let's stretch your low back and spine as we try to return it to an "S" shape instead of the rounded "C" shape. Imperfect sitting conditions have made you sit so your spine looks more like the letter "C" when it should look more like an "S." This puts added stress on areas you don't want to stress. This stretch also helps keep the fluids of the body moving. Please do this healthy stretch slowly three times, holding for 15 seconds.

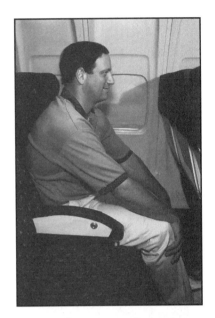

Photo 10-9. Sit slightly forward in your seat with your knees slightly apart. Put your hands on your knees.

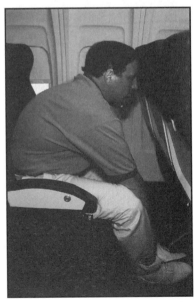

Photo 10-10. I'm rounding my back to stretch out all the muscles as I slide my hands down to my ankles. Do this stretch slowly and enjoy the stretching feeling.

Landing Gear Up

Stretching Strategies
I think it's a good idea to do these healthy stretches as soon as you can after takeoff. Repeat them throughout the flight to avoid getting stiff and to ensure a peppy attitude when you reach your destination. If you like to sleep, do some healthy stretching before closing your eyes and you'll feel nice and relaxed.

This is an easy, convenient way of stretching the back of your legs, the hamstrings, without getting up out of your seat. Do this stretch three times, alternating legs, and hold for 15 seconds.

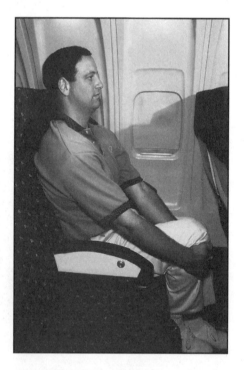

Photo 10-11. Reach down and grab one knee with both hands.

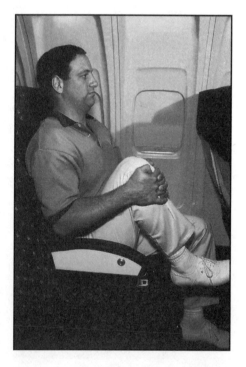

Photo 10-12. Pull your knee slowly toward your chest with your hands. You'll feel the stretch in the back of your legs up through your derrière.

Highway Prisoners

Many of us spend a continuous hour or more commuting back and forth to work, chauffeuring the kids around, or just doing errands. If you live in a large metropolitan area, you may spend even more time captured in your car. Even with all the audio equipment and books on cassette, it's still a Mr. Stretch "TPS," or tension-producing situation.

If you drive long distances for business, or enjoy taking vacations where you are confined to the car for long periods of time, you're a captured commuter too. Unlike the run-of-the-mill sitter, captured commuters are confined to extremely small spaces without the ability to move around freely. Sitters can rotate in their chairs and get up briefly, but you can't do that. Using a friend's convertible, for ease of demonstration purposes, I'll show you how to do some healthy stretching along the way.

> **Chris's Concerns**
> While passengers can do these stretches anytime while traveling, drivers shouldn't—for safety reasons. If you're stuck in a traffic jam or parked in a rest area, turn the car off before starting any of these healthy stretches.

Steering-Wheel Twist

Let's begin by stretching out your upper back. It's also a good stretch to prepare your arms in case a sudden turning of the wheel is needed. Repeat three times and hold for 15 seconds. Taking a deep breath as you hold the stretch helps relieve tension.

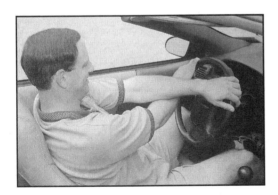

Photo 10-13. Crisscross your arms placing them on opposite sides of the steering wheel. Keep your back straight against the seat but bring your shoulders forward. You'll feel them stretching.

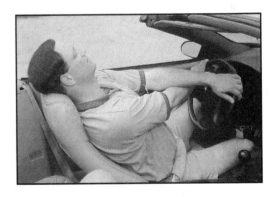

Photo 10-14. Stretch your head back as your shoulders are going forward. This provides a healthy stretch between your shoulder blades and in the front of your chest.

Door Stretch

Using the door will help you stretch away some tension from your upper body. If you've been a little tense from working all day, driving home in a traffic jam is not usually a fun-filled experience. This healthy stretch can help. Do this stretch before you start your trek homeward. Use the door on one side and repeat for the other side, using a seat for leverage. Hold for 15 seconds and repeat two or three times on each side.

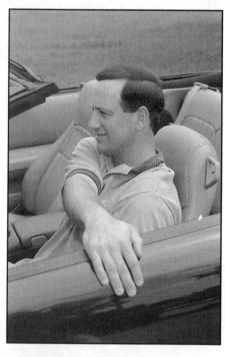

Photo 10-15. Sitting with your shoulders against your seat, reach across your body and grab the door.

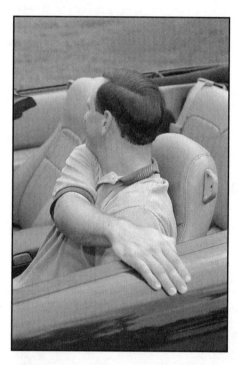

Photo 10-16. Look away from your hand slowly and you'll feel the stretch in your neck and along your arm.

Head-Rest Arm Stretch

This healthy stretch gets your arms above your head as it stretches out your shoulders and upper back. Be sure to do this stretch while stopped, with the engine turned off or in park. Hold for 15 seconds as you stretch three times.

You Heard What?

If you've heard that adjustable car seats should be tilted back to protect against back problems, that's not correct. A tilted back position forces your body to become rounded like a "C" as your hands hold the wheel. This can create some lower back discomfort. When driving, you should adjust your seat as upright as you can to provide a firm feeling of support for your lower back.

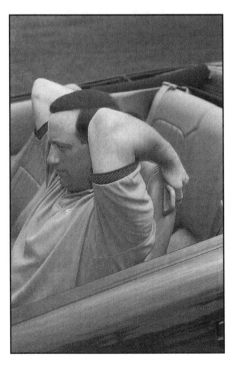

Photo 10-17. Reach over your head and place your hands on the head rest.

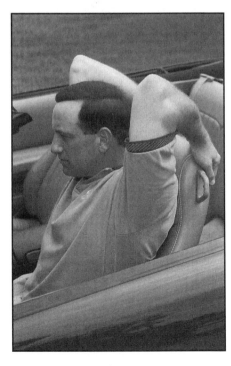

Photo 10-18. Stretch your head and shoulders slowly forward as far as you can.

One-Arm Seat Stretch

Constantly bending your arms as you hold the steering wheel calls for some healthy stretching to lengthen the muscles. Try this stretch whenever you take a break during a long drive.

You'll feel the stretch in your elbow and through your arm. To stretch the other arm, place it on the outside of the door and hold on for leverage as you stretch toward the inside of the car. Repeat three times for each arm, holding for 15 seconds.

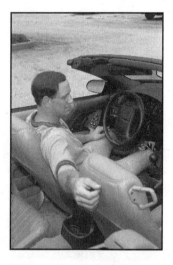

Photo 10-19. Extend your arm behind the passenger seat.

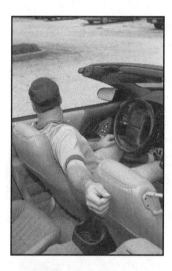

Photo 10-20. Turn and stretch slowly in the opposite direction.

Lumbar Roll Stretch

As you sit for long periods of time, your lower back gets tired. This healthy stretch is similar to some of the stretches you did earlier when you arched and lowered your back. Since you're in a car and can't get down on all fours to feel the benefits, this in-your-seat stretch will still stretch the back muscles. Hold each position for about five seconds before slowly changing your spine angles.

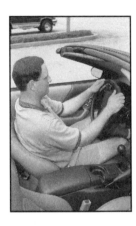

Photo 10-21. Sitting up straight, grab the steering wheel with both hands.

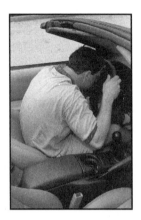

Photo 10-22. Round your back so you can stretch out the muscles. I've touched my head to the steering wheel.

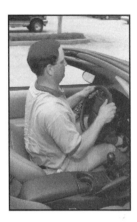

Photo 10-23. Straighten your back slowly as much as you can. You've now stretched your spine in two directions.

Accelerator Stretch

If you're sitting in your car for a long time, your hamstrings, the large muscles in the back of your thighs, are going to get really tight. Not a comfortable situation. At your earliest opportunity, when the car is turned off, I would like to have you give them a healthy stretch. Hold each leg for 15 seconds and repeat one or two times.

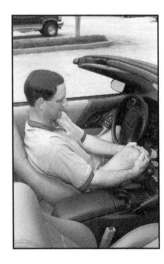

Photo 10-24. Reach down and grab your knee with both hands.

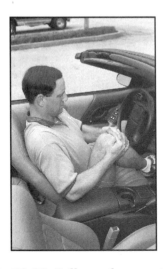

Photo 10-25. Pull your knee up toward your chest. You'll feel the stretch in the back of your thigh and into your derrière.

151

Mr. Stretch Knows Best

I hope you now believe that healthy stretching can blend in to your lifestyle without taking a lot of time. And the more familiar you become with the stretches, the easier it will be to recognize when you can do them.

Please try to do some healthy stretching before any situation where your muscles are going to have limited movement. If you're waiting to board a plane, do some in the lounge area. If you're driving, do some before you start out and during breaks in the trip.

In addition to the healthy stretches I've demonstrated in this chapter, you may want to blend in some of the stretches in Chapter 8 designed for sitters. Healthy stretching allows you to put together the stretches you feel are most effective for you. I suggest changing your selection occasionally to make sure all affected muscles groups get some help.

All of the healthy stretches in this chapter can also be done in a bus or train. Although you won't have a steering wheel, you'll find you can adapt them to fit your needs. If you're waiting for a cab, don't hesitate to sneak a few in. A good one for a Curbside Commuter is the heel drop. Stand on the curb with your heels extended past the pavement. Simply lower one heel at a time slowly and hold for 15 seconds to refresh your legs. You may be a Captured Commuter, but at least your muscles can be free.

The Least You Need to Know

➤ Healthy stretch your muscles before and during a trip to maintain your flexibility.

➤ Airline seats make ideal stretching machines.

➤ Remove your wallet if you're planning on sitting for long periods of time.

➤ Stretching in your car will keep you alert and safe and reduces tension.

Part 4
Good Sports: Mr. Stretch's Program for Flexibility

It's true that some of my sports clients have won baseball's Cy Young Award and several major championships in golf since we began working together. I'm not taking a bow for their success—instead, it is my belief that healthy stretching allowed them to be able to make the changes and improvements their coaches wanted.

You'll find that healthy stretching will also help prevent injuries while conditioning your muscles so you can perform better. After all, I want you to be one of Mr. Stretch's new and improved Weekend Warriors.

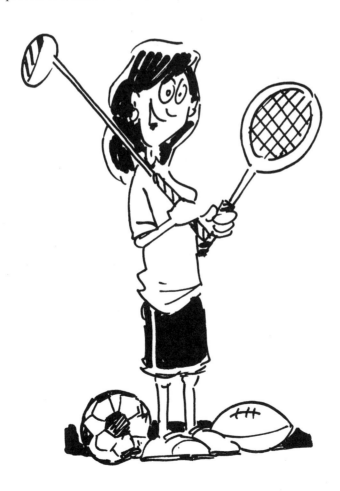

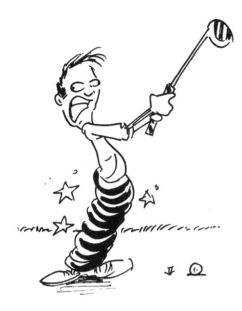

Chapter 11

Golf: Rotating All the Way to the Hole

In This Chapter

➤ Is your golf instructor asking you to make swing corrections your body can't hold?

➤ Consistently hitting good shots requires joint flexibility

➤ Using a golf cart for more than transportation

➤ Improving your golf scores

> The stretches I do every morning ensure a healthy golf day
> —Nick Faldo, three-time Masters Champion

I'm not taking the credit for all the major championships or PGA tournament victories that my clients win. However, healthy stretching allows them to make the swing changes their coaches, like David Leadbetter, request.

If you've been to golf academies or taken lessons from your club pro, do you ever wonder why, when practicing alone, you can't consistently master what you've worked on? It's not always your fault! Instructors may have asked for positions and swing changes your body's just not flexible enough to adapt to. So you revert, bit by bit, back into your old habits.

Pros have the same problem. Sometimes their swing coaches ask them to make adjustments they can't master consistently; being consistent is the hallmark of a top money winner. What's the problem you have in common with some of the best known pros in the game? *Rotational flexibility*, but to understand it better, think of it as joint flexibility.

You Heard What?

"You'll get used to it. It's unnatural at first." Ever heard those phrases from your instructor? They're wrong—you won't get used to it. As instructors watch, they'll correct you when you're creeping back into old swing positions. When practicing by yourself, muscles revert back to the path of least resistance because they're not flexible enough to consistently hold the new positions. The bad shots return.

I've been working with PGA teaching sections around the country, helping identify these problems. Soon you may be surprised when your pro suggests some healthy stretches along with swing corrections.

Rotational Golf

Golf's a totally rotational sport that requires joint flexibility. Your golf swing is a *compilation of compensations* reflecting your flexibility and strength problems. Most of the problems occur during the backswing, as joint tightness invites compensation when you're taking the club back. Just getting back to the ball requires making all sorts of power- and accuracy-robbing swing adjustments. Look at your swing on video and you'll see what I mean. If one muscle's supposed to do a certain job but the joint is tight, another muscle may be compensating to do the work of that muscle. On video the swing looks jerky and off balance.

The golf swing should be, in the words of the legendary Alex Morrison, "one free-flowing motion, unencumbered by physical or mental interruption." Is that how your swing looks?

The way the body moves dictates whether swing plane and ball flight will be correct before contact with the ball is even made. By looking beyond obvious technique problems, golf instructors need to consider the compensations students are making because of a lack of flexibility. If you're the student, the compensation has to be corrected before you can swing correctly. Here is some more interesting information:

➤ Flexibility allows joints to cock and uncock naturally, increasing clubhead speed.

➤ Clubhead speed makes the ball go farther. Swinging hard at the ball doesn't create clubhead speed.

➤ Develop more clubhead speed by allowing the club to swing naturally through the ball—don't steer it.

➤ Power in the golf swing comes from the big muscles of the body.

➤ Healthy stretching improves balance, allowing you to address the ball properly.

➤ Healthy stretching smaller muscles, like the hip flexor muscle group, helps provide support to the big muscles, enabling them to perform.

Golf Carts: More than Transportation Around the Course

Although this Guide is not about golf instruction, healthy stretching for a few minutes before you start playing can improve your game. Hips, knees, and shoulders can be stretched using the golf cart. If you're not taking a cart, benches work just as well.

It's just as important to do the same stretches after you've played, too. Think of your score as rotations. Double that number—since you swing the club in both directions, up and back. That's not even counting practice swings or bending to tee up your ball, replace divots, and remove the ball from the hole. You've used your muscles to rotate through the round and they've become fatigued and shortened. Taking a few extra moments will stretch them back to their normal range. You'll feel a lot better and avoid some stiffness. The 19th hole can wait a few more minutes.

Cart Quad Stretch

Power in your golf swing comes from the big muscles in your legs, like the quadriceps in the front of your thighs. Their unwinding, as the downswing begins, helps create powerful centrifugal force and clubhead speed. Feel the slow stretching of the quads and hold for 15 seconds. Alternate legs and do this healthy stretch three times.

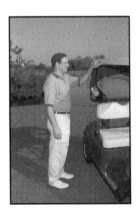

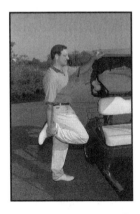

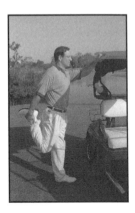

Photo 11-1. Face the side of the cart placing one hand on the roof for balance.

Photo 11-2. Bring one foot back and hold in front of the ankle with your hand that's on the same side.

Photo 11-3. Stretch your heel slowly toward your derrière or as far as it can go, feeling the stretch in the front of your bent leg. Try to gently stretch farther each time.

157

Birdie Hip Stretch

This healthy stretch will increase your hip rotation. You'll be able to turn back from the ball on the backswing and finish facing your target. Do the stretch gently but firmly and work toward trying to get your crossed leg as flat as you can.

It's very important to also do this stretch just after finishing your round. Hold the two stretch positions for 15 seconds, then change legs. After you've stretched each hip once, notice which knee of the crossed leg seemed to be higher. When you repeat the stretch, do that leg three times and your other leg twice to help equalize them.

Photo 11-4 (Left). Sit on the passenger side of the golf cart.

Photo 11-5 (Right). Cross one leg over the other so your ankle rests on your thigh. The crossed knee will be higher if you're not flexible and flatter if you are.

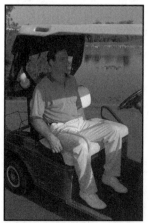
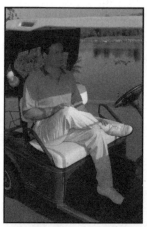

Photo 11-6 (Left). Push gently but firmly down on the crossed knee. You'll feel the stretch on the outside of the hip where it meets your leg. Hold for 15 seconds.

Photo 11-7 (Right). To increase the stretch, slowly lean forward. You should immediately feel additional stretching. Hold for 15 seconds.

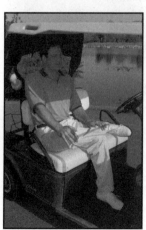
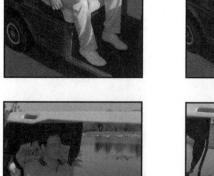
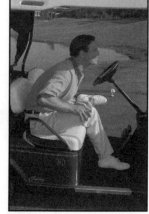

Eagle Inner Thigh Stretch

Muscles of the inner thigh are a group most people don't even think about, until they strain them. It's important to balance the leg muscles by doing these healthy stretches as you prepare the power engines of your swing, the legs, for the round ahead. Repeat three times, holding for 15 seconds, and alternate legs for each stretch. This also allows you to become aware of your body's flexibility and to determine which muscles need additional healthy stretching.

Chris's Concerns
If you know you have a hip problem that has required a doctor's care, please do not do the Birdie Hip stretch. If you develop any sharp pains, stop immediately. Recheck the demonstration. If you did it correctly, some other problem may be contributing to your limited flexibility and you should consult your doctor.

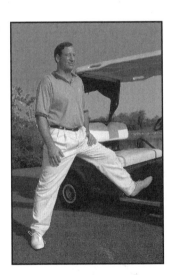

Photo 11-8. Begin by standing to the side of your cart facing forward. Raise the closest leg to the cart and, keeping it straight, place your heel in the cart.

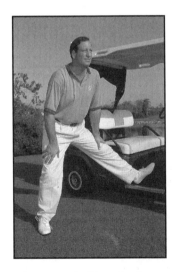

Photo 11-9. Keep both legs straight as you place your hands on your thighs.

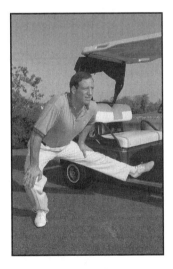

Photo 11-10. Slowly lower yourself down as you bend the knee of the leg you are standing on. You'll feel the stretch, believe me, on the inside of your raised leg's thigh.

159

Long Driver Shoulder Turn

Many recreational golfers have *arm-dominated swings,* meaning they use mostly their arms to swing at the ball. The pros use hip turns followed by big shoulder turns on the backswing, winding up their bodies. When they start their downswing, it's actually releasing all of this energy as the club starts back toward the ball. Longer drives are the result. Compare that with an amateur's locked-hip, small-shoulder movement.

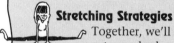
Stretching Strategies
Together, we'll get your body ready for power golf, but you may need some other help. Your local pro can take your new found flexibility and put it to good use. Champions still take lessons.

This healthy shoulder stretch will loosen up the big muscles of your shoulder. Working together with the big muscles of the legs, a powerful force can be unleashed and your ball will sail well beyond your normal landing area. Hold both stretch positions for 15 seconds and then alternate shoulders by changing your golf cart position. If you were facing forward, turn around to face the back. Please do this healthy stretch three times slowly.

Stand in a good athletic position sideways to your cart. Your hands should be on your knees as you lean forward.

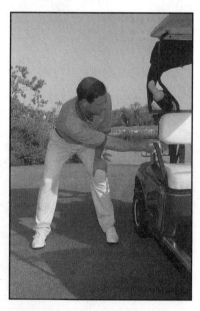

Photo 11-11. Reach across and, with your outside arm, grasp the cart's seat rest.

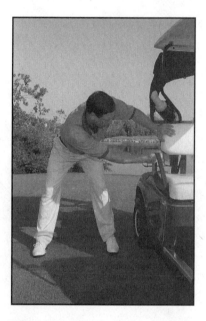

Photo 11-12. Place your other hand toward the top of the seat.

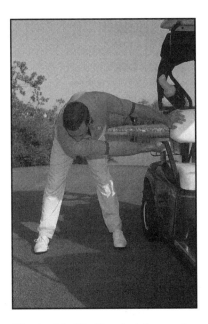

Photo 11-13. To stretch, gradually push your top hand while pulling the bottom hand. You'll feel your shoulders slightly rotate and stretch. Hold for 15 seconds.

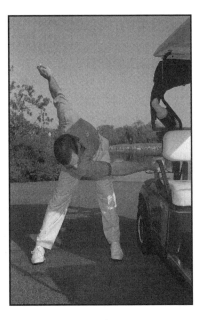

Photo 11-14. Release your top hand off the seat, slowly rotating it to a vertical position or as far as you can comfortably go. Hold for 15 seconds.

This stretch should be done slowly. Feel the muscles stretch. It's especially important to stretch slowly to the final position, going only as far as you can comfortably hold for 15 seconds. The vertical position should be your goal, but if you can't reach it, you're still increasing your own range of motion as you stretch.

You Heard What?

If anyone ever told you to keep your back straight and your head down when you address the ball, they were wrong. The spine is not designed to be straight. The spine is designed to be an "S" curve.

Look at Lisa's address position in Photo 11-15. Mentally draw a straight line from the back of her head to the base of her spine. See how the spine naturally curves in at her neck and lower back. Her head's not pointing down at all. It's easier to hit consistent shots from an address position that's balanced and flexed.

Address for Success

Golf's a mental game, so think positively at all times. As you do these healthy stretches before your round, visualize how you want to play the first hole. The ball flies off your driver, climbs and streaks down the fairway, landing in perfect position. You fade your second shot over two cavernous bunkers, landing softly on the green. Your 10-foot birdie putt starts to the right and then makes the break you read, dropping into the hole.

Maintaining good posture, in the address position, is vitally important if you want to consistently hit good golf shots. How can you be consistent if your body has to make compensations just to have you stand up to the ball?

Photo 11-15. Lisa is in a good athletic position.

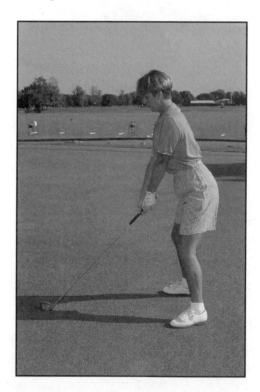

Great golf instructors, like David Leadbetter, believe you should be in a good athletic position at address. In Photo 11-15, Lisa is well balanced, flexed, and ready to make good hip and shoulder turns. The big muscles of her body are ready, willing, and able to make a good golf swing.

Stretch for a Rotational Swing

Rotate the hips and shoulders to lower your scores. The ball should go straighter and longer if you allow centrifugal force to take over. Don't steer the shot. Trust your muscles and joints while making flexible turns for better golf. This rotational golf swing stretch is something you may want to do during your whole round. It educates the muscles to rotationally move through the golf swing. Do it slowly and hold the backswing and follow-through positions for 15 seconds. Repeat two or three times.

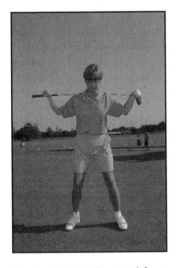

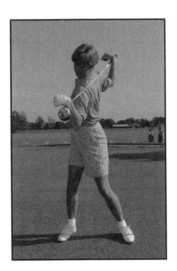

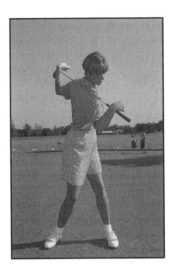

Photo 11-16. Start with a good athletic position, knees flexed, club on your shoulders. Wrap your wrists around the top of the shaft so they are more towards each end.

Photo 11-17. Rotate and stretch into the backswing position. Try and stretch so the grip portion of the shaft points past the ball.

Photo 11-18. Slowly rotate back around to the follow-through position. Feel your back and hips stretch.

The Least You Need to Know

➤ You must rotate with your joints in order to hit the golf ball effectively.

➤ The big muscles of your body create the power—keep them flexible.

➤ Your spine was designed to be an "S" curve, not straight.

➤ If you want to be consistent and improve, healthy stretch your way to flexibility.

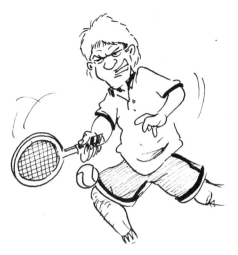

Chapter 12

Tennis: Love the Flexibility

In This Chapter

➤ What every muscle needs to know about tennis

➤ Avoiding injuries by preparing the muscles to play

➤ Some healthy stretches to avoid tennis elbow

➤ Stretching protection for your Achilles tendon

Tennis is a sport featuring quick bursts of energy followed by periods of rest. Your heart rate goes up and down to match the energy requirements. If you could chart your heart rate on a monitor, you'd see the spikes where energy was needed and how it returns to normal rates in between. The heart is one muscle I can't help you with. Its muscle tissue is constructed differently and it *contracts and relaxes involuntarily*, which means it works on its own without your conscious help. If I could invent stretches that worked for hearts, perhaps I could write a sequel to this Guide—*The Complete Idiot's Guide to Living Forever*.

Just as your heart rate has to endure quick starts along with quick stops when you play tennis or other racquet sports, so do the muscles of the body. Most people don't realize their whole body is starting and stopping and starting again, creating wear and tear on the muscles and joints. Here's what can happen while you're playing a single point:

➤ You bend unnaturally backward as you toss the ball into the air for your first serve.

➤ Your shoulders, elbow, and wrist rotate around to strike the ball.

➤ Your back and shoulders extend to reach the ball as it descends.

➤ Your shoulders, back, arms, wrists, hips, and knees rotate forward after the ball has been hit, as the body searches for balance.

➤ Unless you aced your opponent, the ball will be returned and you'll have to rotate your ankles, knees, and hips to get within range and probably have to extend your shoulders and arms to get your racket on it.

And all of this takes place in just seconds.

The Weekend Warrior Syndrome

As you've learned throughout the Guide, your muscles may not be ready to jump into action and perform without letting you know they're protesting. At the height of tennis's popularity, lots of people thought it was a nice leisurely activity and didn't prepare themselves. The more they played, injuries like *tennis elbow* set in. Not knowing what caused it led to not knowing how to treat it. People overlooked their minor injuries hoping they would go away, but they didn't. You can't open a can to replace your injured or fatigued muscles with new ones.

In the course of your normal activities, how many times do you put your hands above your head? Unless you're reading this in the county jail, very infrequently. When you go out to play tennis for an hour, you're putting your hands above your head in a repetitive situation. If you never prepare yourself by strengthening for that movement and expect not to get hurt, you're asking for a lot. If you never got hurt playing tennis as a kid, it doesn't mean you weren't creating a problem for yourself later in life.

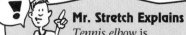

Mr. Stretch Explains

Tennis elbow is actually *tendonitis*, an inflammation of the tendons on the outside of the lower arm caused by a variety of reasons. One reason is using just the arm to hit the ball. The jarring of the elbow as it absorbs all the energy is passed on to the tendons. One way to avoid tennis elbow is to get the body involved with the shot. It helps absorb the shock of energy, while providing power for the return. Make sure you also use a properly weighted and balanced racquet.

Before Lisa demonstrates the healthy stretches I recommend for my professional tennis clients, here's a list of problems tennis players can develop. How many of these have you experienced?

➤ Tennis elbow

➤ Tender wrists

➤ Shoulder problems

➤ Knee and hip problems

➤ Back strains

➤ Shoulder rotation problems

If you're a Weekend Warrior, you've probably experienced the discomfort from quite a few on the list. One of the worst side effects of injuries is they probably kept you from playing the sport you love so much. These healthy stretches should be done before you play and you should select some to do right after your match. Muscles fatigue and shorten with use. Taking a few moments to stretch them back to their normal lengths is another injury preventative measure.

Upper Body Stretches: Stretching From the Top Down

Unlike the stretches for some of the other sports, I prefer to have you begin by stretching for tennis from the top down. It's easier to do and with all the jarring and quick energy bursts ahead of you, it's also relaxing. Healthy stretching before your match will allow you to raise your performance level. Since you can trust your body to perform, knowing it's been properly prepared, your range of motion will be increased and you may be able to go after that cross court shot you've watched sail by in previous matches.

Behind the Back Racket Stretch

This healthy stretch will help the muscle groups used during all parts of the game. It's a nice easy way to start preparing. Please repeat two or three times and hold both stretch positions for 15 seconds, alternating arms.

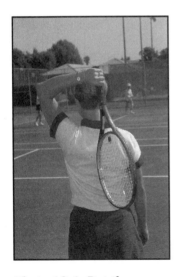

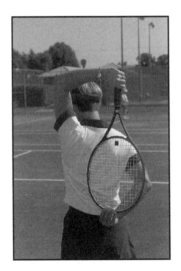

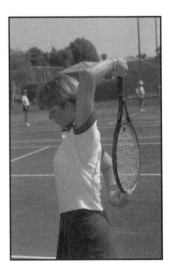

Photo 12-1. Put the racquet behind your head, between your shoulder blades.

Photo 12-2. Reach your other hand back, grasping the racquet. You'll feel the stretch in your arms and shoulders. Hold for 15 seconds.

Photo 12-3. Push your hands away from your body to increase the stretch even more. Hold for 15 seconds.

Under Grip Net Stretch

It's important to keep your wrists and elbows flexible. They have to position the racquet quickly and absorb a lot of energy as the ball rebounds off the strings. This is a healthy stretch designed to help prevent tennis elbow. Repeat three times for each arm, holding for 15 seconds.

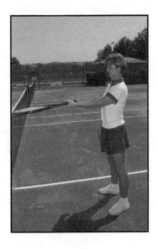

Photo 12-4. Rest the racquet on the net in front of you, holding it from underneath the grip with one hand.

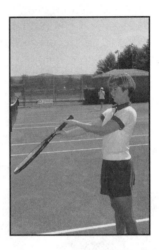

Photo 12-5. Step back as you place your other hand on the lowest portion of the grip. Slightly bend the top elbow as you slowly and very gently pull down with the lower arm.

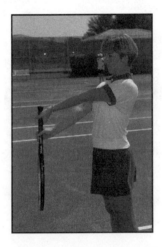

Photo 12-6. Slowly straighten the top elbow for a full stretch of the under part of your lower arm. Hold for 15 seconds.

Avoid Tennis Elbow: Over Grip Net Stretch

Both the Under Grip and Over Grip Net stretches help prevent tennis elbow. This is almost the same stretch as the previous one. The big difference is that you now hold the racquet from the top of the grip as you rest it on the net. You don't need to bend your elbow, so keep the top arm straight. You'll feel the stretch on the top of your wrist. Change arms and repeat three times. Hold for 15 seconds.

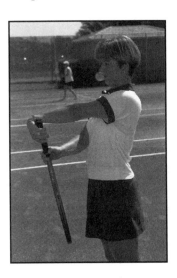

Photo 12-7. This is the 15-second holding position for the Over Grip Net stretch. Compare the hand's position on top of the grip with Photo 12-4 where Lisa is holding it from underneath.

You Heard What?

True or false? If you started tennis as a kid, your body is used to the demands of the sport. False! Because very few people ever take care of themselves as kids, they don't realize that their injuries will appear later in life. The starting and stopping affects the ankles. When ankles are hurt, hips become tight. It's a compensation the body makes to prevent further injury.

Shoulder problems develop over long periods of time. Having trouble getting your serves in may be a symptom of a shoulder problem. Serving requires the ability to extend your arm all the way out while rotating it.

169

Serving Stretches

One of my clients came in and said he had a problem with his second serve. His shoulder was tight, so he couldn't turn his arm properly to get the extra spin on the slower serve. After stretching him, I suggested some healthy stretches for him to do on his own. A month later he came in for a "check-up." When I asked, "How's your second serve?" he answered, "I don't know, Chris, I'm getting my first serve in!"

These healthy stretches may end up surprising your opponent as you ace them. Be sure to do them slowly.

First Serve Stretch

Use the fencing to help stretch your muscles for that killer serve. As you stand with your back to the fence, start with the arm you serve with and do the stretch three times. Stretch your other arm only once. Hold for 15 seconds.

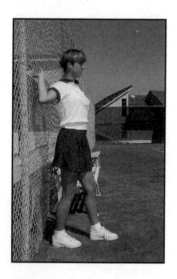 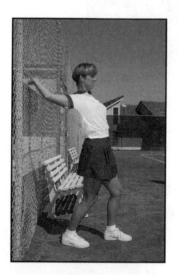 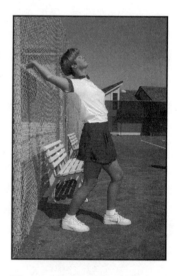

Photo 12-8. Put your hand slightly above your shoulder and reach back to hold one of the fence rings.

Photo 12-9. Step away from the fence so your whole body is extending out from your hips to your shoulders. Your elbow should not straighten.

Photo 12-10. To really feel the stretch, tilt your head back and arch your back. You'll feel it from your hand all the way down to your waist.

Biceps Fence Stretcher

I want you to always include this stretch as part of your pre-match warm-up. In tennis, your arms are usually bent and don't fully extend. You risk developing an overuse syndrome of your biceps. This healthy stretch will help keep you on the court. Stand with your back to the fence and stretch each arm alternately three times, holding for 15 seconds.

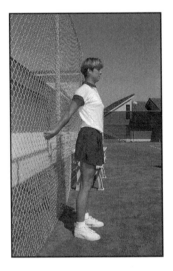 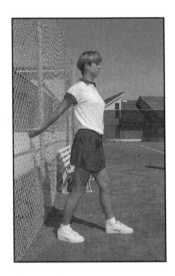 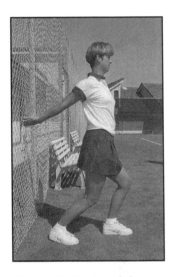

Photo 12-11. Reach your hand back, with your thumb down, grabbing the fence about waist high.

Photo 12-12. Take a step away from the fence. Your shoulder should start to drop down as your arm extends. The stretch should begin at the front of your shoulder to your elbow.

Photo 12-13. Bend down slowly, keeping your shoulders over your hips. This will fully stretch your biceps muscle on the front of your arm.

Legs: The Power of the Game

Your legs have big responsibilities. They have to propel, balance, and position you to reach and hit the ball. Depending on the surface you're playing on, they have to stop quickly or slide into the shot. I guess we had better get to work preparing them. These are basic leg healthy stretches. Lisa will also demonstrate some leg stretches for sliding surfaces in the next section.

Ankle Stretcher

This healthy stretch prepares the muscle groups from the ankles up to the inner thigh. Done properly, it can help protect you from *Achilles tendon* injuries, named after the Greek warrior who was killed in the battle of Troy when a spear struck the only vulnerable part of his body, his heel. The Achilles tendon connects the calf to the heel and usually requires surgery when it becomes torn.

Use the edge of the court where it meets the fence. Alternate legs and hold for 15 seconds in both stretch positions.

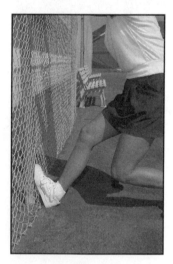

Photo 12-14. Put your heel as close as you can to the fence. The closer it is, the more you may have to squat down just to begin.

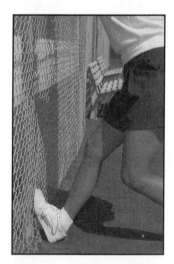

Photo 12-15. Straighten your leg very slowly and increase the stretch as you raise up toward the fence. You'll feel the stretch in the back of your leg. Hold for 15 seconds.

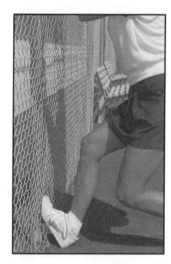

Photo 12-16. Bend your knee to get some other muscles involved in the stretch, the ones located in front of your calf. Hold for 15 seconds.

Standing Quad Stretch

The quads, the big muscles in front of your thighs, are extremely important in tennis. They create the power you need to play effectively. Alternate legs, holding the stretched position for 15 seconds. Stretch each leg three times.

To really prepare the quads, stretch slowly as you try to touch your heel to your derrière. Your knee should pass your hips but your shoulders should not dip forward. If you can't comfortably reach your derrière, get closer to the fence as you hold the stretch during each repetition.

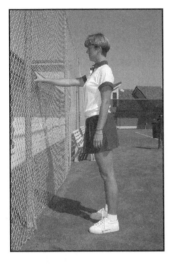

Photo 12-17. Stand facing the fence or the net placing one hand on it.

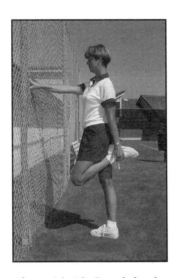

Photo 12-18. Reach back and grab one foot as you bend your knee.

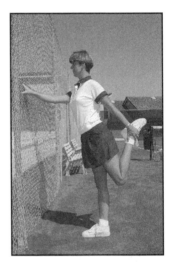

Photo 12-19. Slowly pull your knee back, feeling the stretch in the front of your thigh as you try to touch the heel to your derrière.

173

Chris's Concerns

When doing this hamstring stretch, the temptation is to put your toes up. Do not, I repeat, do not do this. People injure themselves doing their own stretches thinking they are making their calves feel better by putting the toe up. The problem is, if you have back problems, the hip can be affected. So keep your foot as flat as you can.

Bench Stretch Your Hamstring

In tennis, you're always bending and flexing and your hamstrings take the brunt. Use a bench and repeat three times for each leg, holding for 15 seconds.

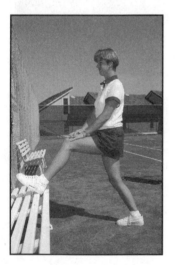

Photo 12-20. Put one foot on top of the bench, knee bent. Keep your back straight.

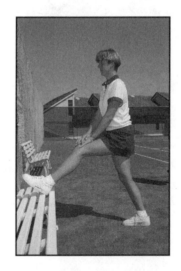

Photo 12-21. Still standing straight, slightly straighten your leg.

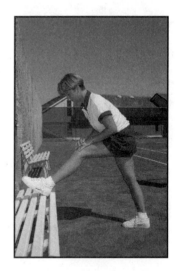

Photo 12-22. Slowly lean forward, keeping your back straight. You'll feel the stretch in the back of your thigh.

Sliding Stretches

These two healthy stretches help you prepare the legs for sliding into shots on clay or similar surfaces. Professional athletes get hurt because they take sliding for granted. As a "Mr. Stretch's new and improved Weekend Warrior," please do these stretches so that you will still have a spring in your step on Monday. Hold each stretch position for 15 seconds.

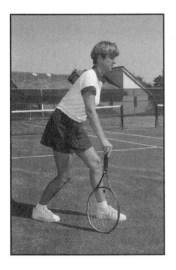

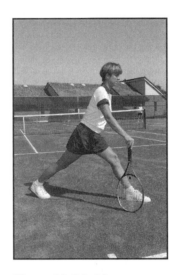

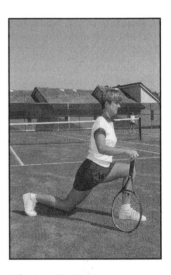

Photo 12-23. Put your racquet on the court for balance. Place one foot slightly behind the other, knees bent.

Photo 12-24. Move your back leg as far back as you can. You'll start to feel the stretch in your back leg.

Photo 12-25. Lean your hips and shoulders forward so your front knee bends but stays over your foot and shoulders remain over your hips. It's okay to keep your back leg bent if you feel the stretch. If you don't, straighten the back leg slowly.

175

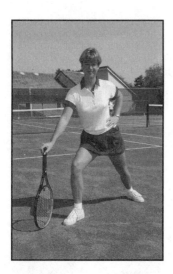

Photo 12-26. This inner thigh version of the sliding stretch is done the exact same way, except your back foot is turned sideways while the leg remains straight.

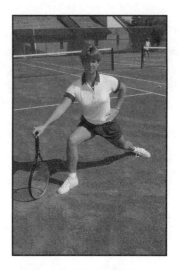

Photo 12-27. In this holding position, the inner thigh of the back leg is being stretched. Hold for 15 seconds.

The Least You Need to Know

➤ You can't open a can and replace your used muscles.

➤ Do some of the stretches immediately after you play, returning fatigued tennis muscles back to normal length.

➤ Stretch slowly, feeling the healthy stretching of your vulnerable tennis muscles.

➤ Tennis requires healthy stretching if you want to raise your performance levels.

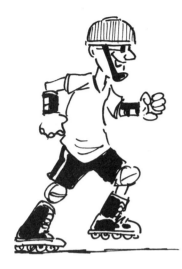

Chapter 13

Leg Sports: Walking, Rollerblading, Cycling, Running, and Climbing

In This Chapter

➤ Participation in these sports means you may be in good shape, but not flexible

➤ Awareness of potential injuries may help prevent them

➤ Weekend Warriors can prevent VCIF—vicious cycle of inflexibility

If you participate in any of the sports that are in this chapter, I'm glad you stopped by. You really like to exercise and, as a result, are probably in pretty good shape. Your sport takes you to see interesting places: spectacular scenic areas, the great outdoors, vast mountain ranges, your doctor's ceiling.

Couldn't slip that one by you? I know you have some solid opinions on how to prepare for leg-dominated sports and you might think stretching isn't necessary. You'll get loose naturally, by taking it easy in the beginning. Want to answer a quick question for me? Please circle the number of the correct choice below.

When stretching your legs, it's important to:

1. Only stretch the muscles in front of your legs.

2. Only stretch the muscles in back of your legs.

3. Stretch just the hamstrings and the quads.

4. Stretch the muscles in the front and back of your legs.

5. Take off and hope for the best.

May I have the envelope please? The answer most leg athletes would incorrectly give, since for the most part it's the only group of muscles I see them stretch, is number #2— the muscles in the back of their legs. The correct answer is #4—stretch the muscles in front *and* back of your legs. Unfortunately, most runners think that by touching their toes, they're stretching both.

You Heard What?

If you've heard that when you participate in leg-dominated exercises it's only important to stretch the muscles in the back of your legs, it's a misconception. Most people believe that stretching means bending over and touching their toes. However, that only stretches the muscle groups in back of the legs. If you don't balance the front and back of the leg muscle groups, the unstretched quads, in the front, get tense, which can create a back problem. That's bewildering to people who say, "But I can touch my toes." That's a good indication that their hamstrings, in the back of the thigh, are stretched, but their quads, in the front of the thigh, aren't.

How the Natural Runners Stretch

If you don't think a few healthy stretches are necessary to prepare your body for leg-dominated sports, let's take a look at the great natural runners. Earlier I mentioned my friend and co-author Steve Hosid's Borzoi hounds, two incredible athletes. They're 6 feet 2 inches high standing up on two feet and stretching their front legs out. Originally bred for chasing and killing wolves, these guys are friendly and very tame. You've probably seen the breed featured in ads for Vodka or jewelry, as they look very aristocratic. But they run very fast, 42 miles per hour, and can change direction on a dime.

What do you think is the first thing they both do when they know it's time for a walk or run? Falcon and Misha both arch their backs, stretching their back muscles. Then they lower their front paws as they raise their rear quarters up, stretching their necks as well as front and rear leg muscles. I didn't teach them that, nature did. Dogs and large cats like jaguars, cheetahs, and other fast predators naturally stretch before they move quickly. Nature instilled in them the basics of injury prevention. Pulled muscles mean they can't run down their prey and satisfy their food demands.

Other animals also stretch. In some cases, being injured with pulled muscles can result in being selected as dinner by the predator animals. So as you watch the nature shows, remember that the cute stretching the animals do when they wake up from a nap has a purpose. Survival!

What Can Go Wrong

Understanding the reason for some injuries or flexibility problems that you may have experienced may help you avoid them in the future. You're really using your legs, and sometimes an injury to one part of the leg, like a twisted ankle, can create a problem someplace else. For instance, hip joint problems are something I see a lot in those of you who participate in leg sports. Knees are also involved because most of the muscles that connect at the hips also connect at the knees.

Runners: Pounding Away

Runners suffer from hip joint injuries caused by constant impact and jarring, along with rotating around their hip joint. What's sometimes overlooked is that runners can twist an ankle and then keep running on it. Compensations the body has to make to protect the ankle stiffen the hip. Sometimes this also results in a knee problem.

Since you tend to move in a straight line as you run, you're restricting the actual motion of your muscles while you're fatiguing them in a very specific pattern. As a result, a lot of runners will trip and fall if something darts out in front of them. They lose their sense of balance because the muscles that make side-to-side movements aren't being used.

Cyclists: Seated Rotational Movers

Cycling requires incredible rotational movement from an unnatural position. The hip joint really has to be free in order to move efficiently, propelling you along. The tendency to have tight quads and hip flexor muscles sometimes creates flexibility problems that can worsen without healthy stretching. Knee injuries can be a result of hip joint inflexibility.

Rollerbladers: Pushing-Off Hip Alert

Just like ice skating, rollerblading requires pushing off with the foot, leg, and hip, which can create deep hip joint flexibility problems. You can develop very tight hip joint muscles that are shortening because they're fatiguing. Just as you protect your body with pads and helmets, protect your hips with some healthy stretching before and after you rollerblade.

Stretching Strategies
Doing some healthy stretches immediately after participating in these leg-dominated sports is extremely important. The workout you put your legs through when you cycle, for example, fatigues the muscles as they use up their stored energy. Healthy stretching lengthens muscles back to their normal length, helping to prevent injury and soreness.

Climbing Machines: Stairways to Tightness

Is this you? You go to the health club and really feel nice and loose while working out—for example, on the climbing machine—but when you cool down later you feel sore and stiff. You can help improve this situation by doing a few healthy stretches before to prepare the muscles for the exercise, as well as after, to stretch out the fatigued muscles. As muscles fatigue, they shorten and stiffen.

Weekend Warriors: The Vicious Cycle of Inflexibility

As you know, I'm leading the crusade against unneeded stiffness. Here's my rallying cry:

Will you join and stretch with me, as I keep you loose and free?

Healthy stretching will help you avoid *VCIF, the vicious cycle of inflexibility*. This occurs because you sit most of the week and your muscles become shorter. When you go out running, cycling, rollerblading, or whatever, you're fatiguing the already shortened muscles. So you've shortened them due to lifestyle, then shortened and fatigued them from activity. When you go to work the next day and sit again, usually uncomfortably, you're in *the vicious cycle of inflexibility*.

Mr. Stretch's Flexibility Favorites

Stretching Strategies
As you stretch your calves to help your Achilles tendon, do it very slowly so you can feel the stretch. Never force the muscle—stretch it instead. Since you're doing several repetitions, try to go a little farther each time. Go only as far as you can, to improve your own range of flexibility.

As a "Mr. Stretch's new and improved Weekend Warrior," your muscles stay healthily stretched at proper lengths. Your muscles are prepared to help you enjoy your leisure time activity and still feel good the next day. I'll demonstrate some healthy stretches to maintain and increase your flexibility.

Calves Pole Stretch

For a runner, calves are the number one tight muscles that usually are overlooked. You want your calves to be stretched in order to avoid tearing the attached Achilles tendon. If you've ever experienced a sharpness of pain in the back of your lower leg above the heel, it's usually from the Achilles tendon. This healthy stretch should be repeated two or three times for both legs. Hold the stretch for 15 seconds.

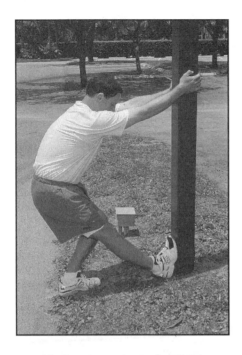

Photo 13-1. Standing close to a pole or small tree, put one heel as close to it as you can. The tighter you are, the lower your derrière will have to go to get your heel close to the pole. Hold the pole in both hands.

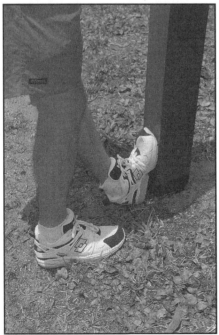

Photo 13-2. Slowly and gently stand up to a point where you really feel the muscle stretching.

Hamstring Striding Stretch

Leg-dominated sports require extending your legs. Balanced muscles working together accomplish this goal efficiently. You've just stretched your calves, which attach above the knee, so now let's stretch the hamstrings, which attach below the knee. Both muscle groups have to be stretched if you want flexible knees.

Use a slightly elevated stone or curb. You want your foot to be below your knee or waist. Repeat twice for each leg, holding for 15 seconds.

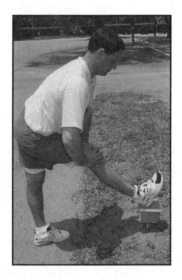

Photo 13-3. As you place one heel on an elevated object, your back foot should be pointing toward your front foot. Place your hands on the knee of the raised leg and keep your back straight over it.

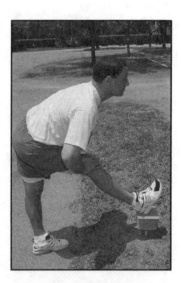

Photo 13-4. Keep your back straight as you slowly lean forward. You'll feel the stretch in the back of your thigh.

Dynamic Quad Stretch

This is a *dynamic stretch* for the quad muscle. Dynamic stretch means you're putting tension on the muscle while stretching it. This healthy stretch works on the quads, the big muscles in front of your thigh.

Alternate legs and hold the stretch for 15 seconds. I suggest doing this stretch two times.

> **Stretching Strategies**
> The Dynamic Quad stretch simulates the actual muscle movements for running, hiking, or other leg-dominated sports. While it stretches the quad muscle, it makes some other muscle groups contract, as they would during a stride. So as one group stretches, the other contracts—the source of body movement.

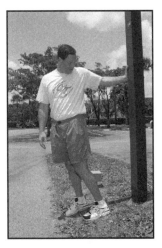

Photo 13-5. Stand with your back to a pole and reach back, holding it with one hand.

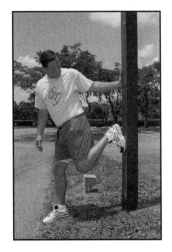

Photo 13-6. Pick up the foot on the same body side as your hand, and reach it back, placing your toes slightly below waist-high on the pole.

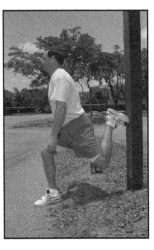

Photo 13-7. Look forward and press your foot against the pole as you push your hips away from the pole.

Inner Thigh Straddle Stretch

The inner thigh muscle, usually associated with moving the leg in and out, is set at an angle to help pick your knee up. If the muscle group is not stretched, it can make the body compensate by adding to the task of the hip flexor muscles. It's like telling your hip flexors it now has two jobs—so it fatigues quicker. The result is you don't feel like running or rollerblading too far. You can also hurt your hip and, if it becomes restricted, back trouble can occur. Have I convinced you to do this healthy stretch yet? Alternate legs and do the stretch two times, holding for 15 seconds.

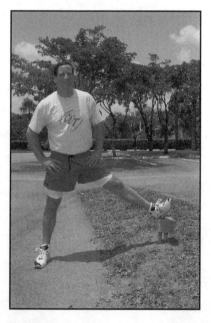 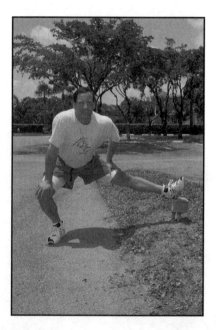

Photo 13-8. Put one foot on an object so that it's higher than the other foot but not as high as your hip. Keep your hands at your sides. Slightly turn out the grounded foot in the direction your knee bends.

Photo 13-9. Slowly stretch to the side but don't allow your knee to go past your grounded foot. You'll feel this in the inner thigh of the straight leg.

Standing Hip Stretch

If you want to run, walk, rollerblade, or move at all, *your hip has to rotate*. This is the best way to stretch your hips standing up. Repeat two or three times for each hip, holding for 15 seconds.

Mr. Stretch Explains
Your hip has to rotate means the femur, the large bone of the upper leg, has to rotate inside the pelvic bone. The top of the femur is shaped like a ball that fits into the socket joint of the pelvis. Since the femur is attached to the hip by various muscle groups, the muscles have to be flexible to allow the femur a free range of motion around the joint.

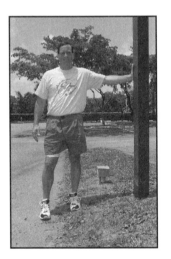

Photo 13-10. Stand sideways to a pole, holding onto it with one hand for balance.

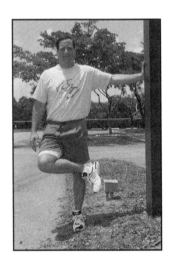

Photo 13-11. Cross one leg over your other knee so that your bent knee is at a 90-degree angle.

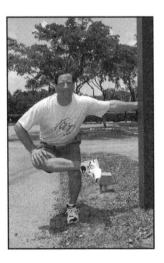

Photo 13-12. Keeping your back straight, bend the standing knee allowing your body to become lower. As your derrière reaches the height of the standing knee, you'll feel the stretch in the bent leg hip joint.

Mr. Stretch Explains

Shin splints is a painful condition of the lower leg. It can be caused by (1) muscles pulling away from the bone or by (2) a stress fracture of the shin bone, or by (3) muscles growing around the bone and putting painful pressure on it. Keeping the muscles stretched will help prevent this situation.

Kneeling Shin Stretch

Let's go back to the legs another time to work on the *shin* muscles of the tibia bone in the lower leg. You may have experienced the discomfort of *shin splints*. This healthy stretch can help prevent this painful condition. I suggest two stretches for each leg, holding for 15 seconds.

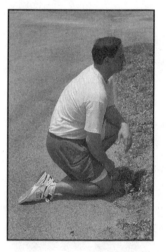

Photo 13-13. Kneel down on one foot with your other leg behind you.

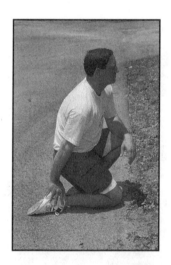

Photo 13-14. Put your same-side hand on your heel and push down. You'll feel the stretch in front of that leg.

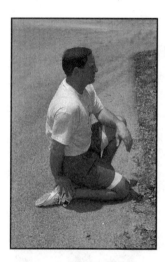

Photo 13-15. If you don't feel the stretch, sit back on your heel and feel the muscle group stretching.

One-Legged Climber Stretch

This is a good healthy dynamic stretch for bikers and rollerbladers as well as climbers. To be a climber, I don't mean you have to mount a major expedition to conquer the north face of Everest. If you like to hike and you're going uphill, try this healthy stretch. Do the stretch one or two times for each leg, holding for 15 seconds.

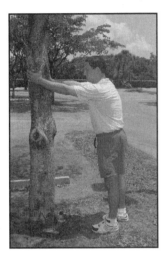

Photo 13-16. Stand about a stride away from a tree and hold it with both hands at shoulder height.

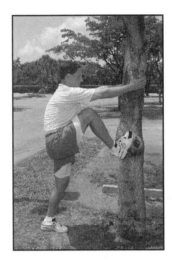

Photo 13-17. I'm pretty flexible so I've put my foot on a knot about waist high. You don't have to go that high.

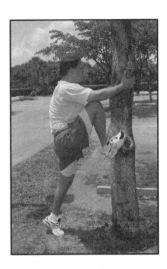

Photo 13-18. Pull your whole body toward the tree. Your hips go forward as your front knee bends. Notice how I'm now standing on my toes. You'll feel the stretch in the front of the raised leg and in the back of the grounded leg.

The Least You Need to Know

➤ It's important to stretch both the front and back muscles of your leg to prevent leg-dominated sports injuries.

➤ Understanding what can go wrong allows you to take steps to prevent flexibility problems.

➤ Healthy stretching will help Weekend Warriors prevent the vicious cycle of inflexibility.

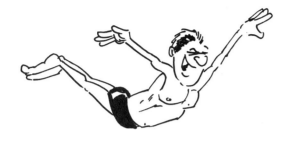

Chapter 14

Swimming: Fluidity in the Water

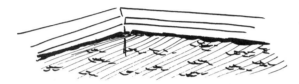

In This Chapter

> ➤ Swimming is often included as therapy for sports-related injuries

> ➤ The swimming "ballet of the joints" promotes muscle harmony

> ➤ Champion athletes have developed body awareness—swimming can help you

> ➤ Swimming requires extended muscles for power

Want to know how perfect a sport swimming is? If you have a sports-related injury, part of your suggested therapy will sometimes include swimming. Even race horses are often sent to aquatic rehabilitation tanks to swim under controlled circumstances.

Water is thought to keep a constant pressure on your body. *Body awareness is extremely important in most sports.* Water pressure helps sharpen that sense. Swimming is a very graceful and controlled-movement sport. But it also requires extremely flexible muscles. Leg-dominated sports like running propel you primarily with the lower portion of the body. Swimming, however, involves the entire body and the variety of strokes requires *various forms of rotation around the joints.* As an example, consider the horizontal shoulder rotations in the breaststroke compared to the vertical rotations in the freestyle.

Swimming Muscle Harmony

Swimming also helps develop coordination between both sides of the body as well as between the opposing muscle groups on the same side. The rhythmical movement creates the great power that propels you through the water. As an example, when swimming freestyle, you may be extending and reaching forward with your right side as your left side is contracting, bringing your hand and arms through the water toward you.

Mr. Stretch Explains

Body awareness is extremely important in most sports. Athletes need to develop a sense and feel for what their bodies are doing. In some cases, it's to regulate and control a certain movement. A pitcher, like John Smoltz, Cy Young Award winner with the Atlanta Braves, needs to feel his front foot touching down after winding up to release his weight and energy, along with his fastball, toward the plate. Michael Jordan can sense his body position even while suspended in the air.

Since you now have a pretty good idea of what healthy stretching is all about, I'm sure you realize a stretched muscle can extend fully and have a greater ability to produce power compared to a muscle that can't extend to its proper length.

The Water Ballet of the Joints

I suggest you do some healthy stretching before swimming to get the most from this wonderful sport. These healthy stretches can also be done at home to really keep the muscles educated for swimming movements. Our first group of stretches will help you develop muscle harmony. This healthy stretch prepares all the muscles of the body and coordinates them before you get in the water. Do it as many times as you like to build your coordination. Hold each position only five seconds.

If you're having trouble holding the positions for these various muscle groups, you may have a strength or flexibility problem. This stretching exercise can help educate your muscles and strengthen them if you rise up, only as far as you can, and hold for five seconds. Each time you do this stretch, try to increase your range of motion.

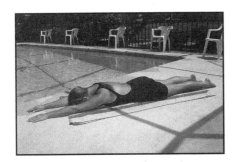

Photo 14-1. Lie face down on a towel, stretching your arms over your head.

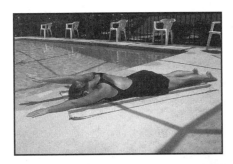

Photo 14-2. Pick up one fully extended arm and hold for about five seconds, feeling the muscles associated with that movement.

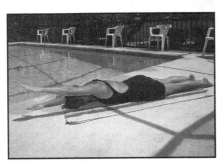

Photo 14-3. Lower it and raise the other arm, creating the same feeling. Hold for five seconds.

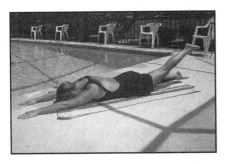

Photo 14-4. Lower the arm and raise one leg as high as you can, keeping it straight. Repeat for the other leg. Hold for five seconds.

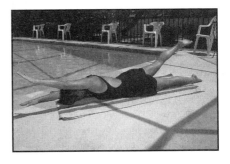

Photo 14-5. Pick up one arm and the opposite leg. You'll feel a crossover stretch across your back in a diagonal motion. Hold for five seconds.

191

Repeat the stretch in Photo 14-5 but change arms and legs. You're developing body awareness as you feel the muscles that will develop the power. Hold the stretch for five seconds, then lower your arm and leg.

Photo 14-6. Starting from the same face-down position, lift up both arms and feel the muscles stretch in your upper back and the tops of your shoulders. Hold for five seconds, then lower them back down.

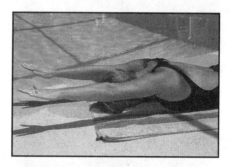

Photo 14-7. Lift up both legs and feel your lower back muscles, the gluteus muscles in your derrière, and your hamstrings stretch. Hold for five seconds, then lower back down.

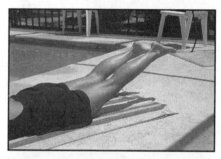

Photo 14-8. Raise both arms and both legs and feel the whole body stretch together. Hold for five seconds.

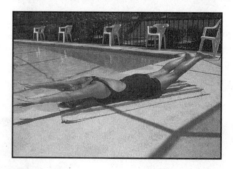

Tuning Up the Engine Stretches

You can spend a lot of time and money making sure a boat's engine is ready to propel you through the water. In swimming, your body is your propeller, rudder, diving planes, and ballast all wrapped up in a bathing suit. As with all the healthy stretches, take your time and feel your muscles slowly stretch.

You Heard What?

If people have told you swimming requires total flexibility, they are wrong. In fact, by stretching the front of their shoulders, many competitive swimmers have hurt themselves. Swimmers need some muscle resistance as a leverage for power. By stretching the front of their shoulders, they can loosen them up too much and create some problems. Swimmers should concentrate on loosening the muscle groups for the back of the shoulders only.

Sleeper Stretch

"Mr. Stretch, you've made our dreams come true; we can stretch while we sleep!" Sorry, I haven't been able to perfect that quite yet. Maybe someday, though. Seriously, the Sleeper stretch uses some of the same positions you should sleep in. Earlier in the Guide I suggested sleeping on your side. This healthy stretch concentrates on the back of the shoulder. Do the stretch three times for each shoulder slowly. Hold for 15 seconds.

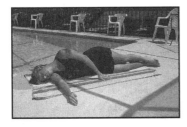

Photo 14-9. Lie on your side, with your lower arm straight out to the side.

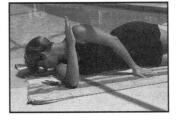

Photo 14-10. Bend the arm to a 90-degree angle at your elbow. Notice how Lisa has put her chin on her shoulder, facing down.

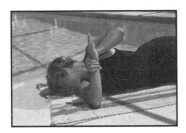

Photo 14-11. Put your opposite hand on the top side of your wrist.

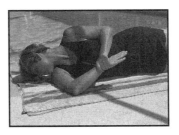

Photo 14-12. Slowly push your wrist toward the ground as you keep your chin on your shoulder. You'll feel the stretch in the back of your shoulder. If you feel it only in the front, adjust your elbow either up or down.

Freestyle Stretch

As you swim freestyle, you generate an upper body twist for power. Use the ladder or some object you can hold onto for this healthy stretch. To stretch the opposite side, face the ladder from the opposite side. Please do this stretch three times per side, holding for 15 seconds.

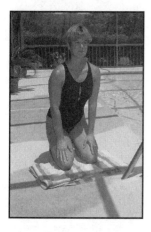

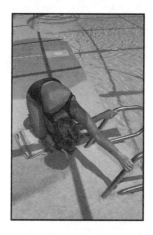

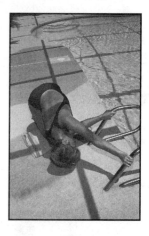

Photo 14-13. With a towel under your legs, sit back on your knees. Lisa is also resting her hands on her knees.

Photo 14-14. Lisa bends down and holds the far rung of the ladder with her extended left hand and the closer portion of the ladder with her crossed-under right hand.

Photo 14-15. To feel the stretch, rotate away from the ladder so there is a straight line from your hip to your left hand. You'll feel the stretch across your body.

Lower Body Power Stretches

The legs are the human version of the tail flipper. As you kick, they propel you through the water. In some cases, like the backstroke, the movements are coordinated with the arms.

Now we're really not capable of competing with water-dwelling mammals in their ability to produce power with our lower body. Let me put it to you this way: If Michael Jordan were appearing at Sea World and had to fly out of the water to grab a fish out of a trainer's hand, he'd starve. On the other hand, out of the water, Flipper's hang time over an NBA rim would be rather limited, too!

Shin Splits Stretch

These healthy stretches work on the legs. Please do them slowly. Lots of recreational swimmers don't realize how much more effective swimming can be when they use their legs.

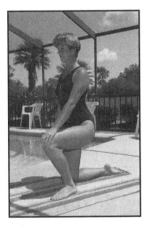

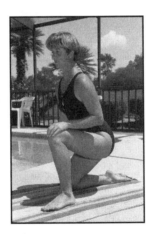

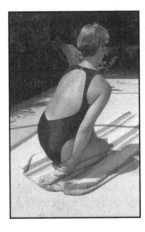

Photo 14-16. Using a towel, kneel on one knee so that your other knee is at a 90-degree angle and your other leg is stretched out behind you.

Photo 14-17. Sit back on your lower leg until you feel the stretch in your shin. If you feel too much stretch, stop where you want to.

Photo 14-18. If you really want to get more of a stretch, this view shows Lisa pushing down gently on her heel, using the hand on the same side.

The Frog

The frog stretch is an excellent healthy stretch for synchronizing the flexibility of your leg movements. It works on just about all the lower body muscles. Lisa will demonstrate it, using a towel to protect her knees. Repeat three times, holding for 15 seconds.

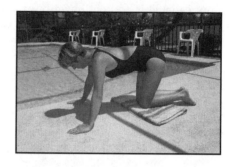

Photo 14-19. Begin on your hands and knees.

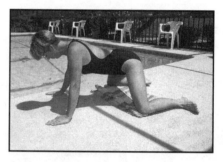

Photo 14-20. Lean forward, keeping your heels and inner parts of your knees touching the ground.

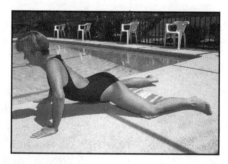

Photo 14-21. Let your hip joints rotate and your pelvis will glide forward as it comes down to the pool deck.

The Least You Need to Know

➤ Swimming is often included as therapy for other sports-related injuries.

➤ The constant pressure of the water helps build body awareness.

➤ Swimming and healthy stretching promote muscle harmony.

➤ Even though swimming is perceived as a gentle sport, your muscles need to be extended and are helped by healthy stretching.

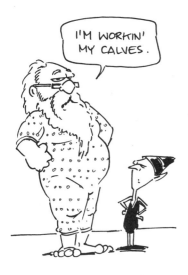

I'M WORKIN' MY CALVES.

Chapter 15

Skiing and Other Winter Sports: Cold-Weather Engine Protection

In This Chapter

➤ Healthy stretching promotes body awareness for winter sports

➤ Preventing injuries on the slopes

➤ Your lower body is a shock absorber

➤ Improving shoulder rotation can improve your skiing

The oldest skis, found in bogs in Finland and Sweden, are thought to be between 4,000 and 5,000 years old. Would you believe it—the bindings still release. Seriously, the skis were elongated curved frames covered with leather. Just think, if you got on a lift line at Aspen 4,000 years ago, you'd almost be at the front of the line now.

Photo 15-1. Healthy stretching can help you enjoy winter sports.

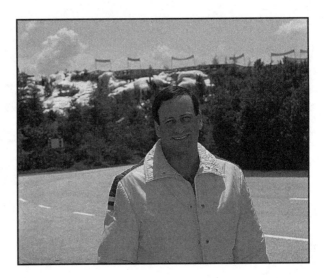

More and more of us are beginning to enjoy winter sports. If you downhill ski, you know the thrill of playing with gravity as you descend the mountain. Cross-country skiing provides some of the best exercise you will ever get. The grace and beauty of ice skating, although not when I do it, is an incredible combination of technique and balance. All of these sports have some obvious differences, but also some similarities. The similarities are what this chapter is about.

Body Awareness

Earlier in Chapter 14, I defined what body awareness is. I think it deserves repeating. All of us need to develop and maintain an awareness of what our body is doing. In some cases, it's needed in order to regulate and control certain movements. For instance, you need to feel the pressure on the bottom of your feet to help maintain balance.

In another fall and winter sport, a football player needs to feel his weight shifting for balance as he dodges and fakes his way through the line. The quarterback needs to feel his body as it coordinates with his brain on how much energy it takes to throw the ball 40 yards compared to 10. Skiers need to be able to feel their bodies react to moguls and also need to feel the weighting and unweighting of their skis necessary for turning. As you carve through the fall line, you have to have a sense of what your body is doing so that you can change your balance and switch edges.

An ice skater needs to have an awareness of what his or her body is doing to time the takeoff for a jump and land correctly. Cross country skiers have to feel their stride and sense differences in terrain in order to adapt quickly. What's happening is that your body is communicating with your brain and making split-second adjustments.

Healthy Stretching Improves Body Awareness

A flexible body is a body that's aware. Flexible joints and muscles can detect differences in terrain and quickly adjust. Flexible muscles can hold positions longer to increase performance. If you were a downhill racer, for example, could you hold the tuck position and change direction quickly if your muscles weren't in shape and prepared to instantly respond?

One of the reasons performance levels of champion athletes have risen so dramatically in recent years is the addition of stretching to their workout routines. For an athlete, having muscles stretched to proper lengths is like tapping into a gold mine. The muscle is longer and that means it has a longer distance to contract, producing added power. Stretched muscles won't fatigue as quickly either, if they're conditioned to maintain their proper lengths.

Asking Santa for Flexibility Doesn't Quite Make it

On a cold winter morning, you usually start your car and let it warm up before driving off. Think of your muscles as the body's engine and warm them up before using them too! You know how stiff a car feels when you first start out; muscles are the same way.

Just bending over in the lift line and doing deep-knee bends doesn't qualify as healthy stretching. Personally, I don't relish the thought of being transported down the mountain by the Ski Patrol and packed off in an ambulance. I'm sure you'd much rather be out enjoying the skiing too! Being able to react to quick changes, while maintaining balance and control, is the key to avoiding injuries. Healthy stretching helps protect you on the slopes. The same is true for all winter sports. The muscles of the body have to be flexible to provide the body awareness so crucial to the sport. I'll be demonstrating some healthy stretching for skiing, but any winter enthusiast will also be able to do them.

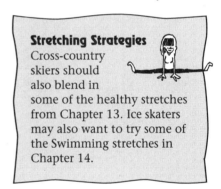

Stretching Strategies
Cross-country skiers should also blend in some of the healthy stretches from Chapter 13. Ice skaters may also want to try some of the Swimming stretches in Chapter 14.

Fall-Line Favorites

Most skiers usually try to get in a nice relaxing run before heading to the moguls. These healthy stretches are a relaxing way to start and should be done before you put on your skis. You may want to do them before putting on your boots. As you stretch, concentrate on what you're feeling—build some body awareness.

When you make your first run, duplicate those feelings. Hold your turns a little longer, allowing the muscles to develop some coordination. Stop and take some deep breaths and relax. As you continue down, concentrate on making rhythmic turns, allowing your body and skis to work together. You'll be aware of the ski releasing its energy and kicking you into the next turn. High-tech skis are expensive; give them a chance to work by preparing your body.

Edge Sharpener

We all know how important it is to keep our skis' edges sharp. This healthy stretch allows your body to sharpen its senses and feel those edges. Do them slowly and feel the edges of your soles as you stretch. Do this stretch twice for each side, holding for 15 seconds.

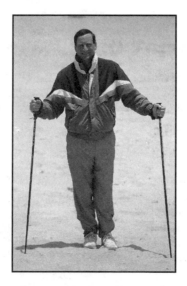

Photo 15-2. Stand up straight with your arms out to your sides holding your ski poles.

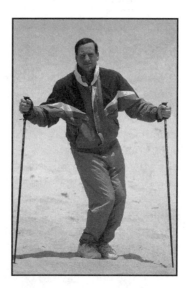

Photo 15-3. Maintaining your straight-ahead position, slowly move your knees to one side.

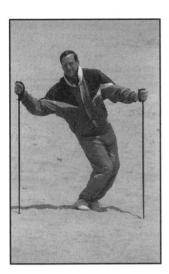

Photo 15-4. Stretch to a position where you start to develop the feeling of edging. You'll feel the stretch in your quads and hip flexors.

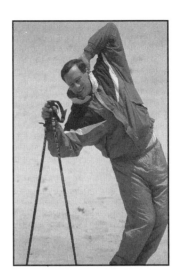

Photo 15-5. Try this stretch after you finish stretching both sides. Plant your poles for support and place one hand on the back of your head. Stretch sideways, bringing your hips to the same side as the raised hand. Hold for 15 seconds and repeat for the other side.

You Heard What?

If you heard that your lower body has to be firm to be a good skier, that's not entirely true. While you want your legs to work together as they weight and unweight, you also want your knees and hips to be flexible.

If you're a beginner or intermediate skier, healthy stretching will help your balance by increasing your body awareness. You don't want to be thrown by quick changes in the terrain. Flexibility allows you to absorb the bumps and change your weighting to keep your skis either edging or running on the snow.

As your body becomes more aware, you'll be surprised at some of the recoveries you can make.

Shock Absorber

Part of maintaining your balance is being able to absorb changes in terrain with your lower body. This healthy stretch works on the "shock absorbers" of the leg—your quads and hamstrings—and also stretches your lower back. Do it slowly and feel the muscles stretching. You'll also need your muscles to be at their proper lengths if you want to get a lot of runs in. Stretched muscles don't fatigue as quickly. The stretch should be done twice, slowly up and slowly down, holding for 15 seconds at the lowest point.

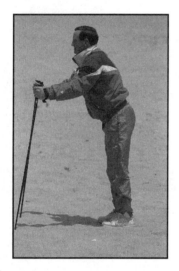

Photo 15-6. Plant your poles in front of you in a position where you have to slightly lean at the waist to reach them.

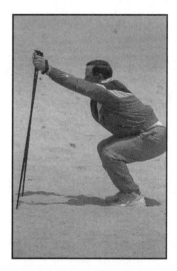

Photo 15-7. Slowly stretch down to a squatting position. If you do this slowly, you will feel your muscles gently stretching.

Mogul Tamers

Your lower body really needs to be in condition if you're off to the mogul fields. Quick changes of direction while absorbing the changes in terrain are what you're asking your muscles to do. If you ski mostly in the Northeast, you'll really have to generate a feeling of holding and releasing your edges with the sometimes icy conditions.

Skiing powder is the ultimate for most skiers. Being able to sit back a little on your skis, unweighting the fronts, helps bring the tips up. These healthy stretches work on the muscle groups you'll need for a long day on the slopes.

Skiers' Quad Stretch

This healthy stretch helps your quads, in front of your thigh, get ready for a heavy day of skiing. If they start to burn and tire as the day progresses, take off your skis and do this healthy stretch. I suggest three times for each leg, holding for 15 seconds.

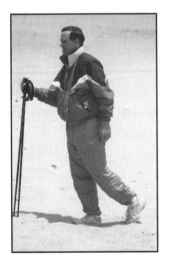
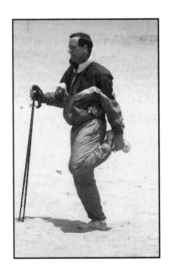
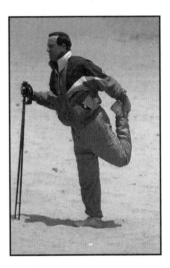

Photo 15-8. Using your poles to keep your balance, start by bringing one foot up toward your back.

Photo 15-9. Reach back and hold your foot, trying to stretch it so it touches your derrière.

Photo 15-10. Slowly stretch your leg back so your thigh and front of your hip feel the stretch.

Skiers' Standing-Hip Stretch

Your hips still need to rotate, even while skiing. Good skiers face down the fall line with their torsos, allowing their lower bodies to rotate and change edges. Since sitting is not exactly a desirable position with your skis on, this is the best way to stretch your hips standing up. Repeat two or three times for each hip, holding for 15 seconds.

If we were skiing together, I'd suggest doing some of these healthy stretches before taking a break in the lodge. As you use your muscles, they shorten from fatigue. A few stretches before going inside will restore their length. Also do a few stretches before starting out again. Taking care of your muscles protects you and will extend your comfortable time on the slopes.

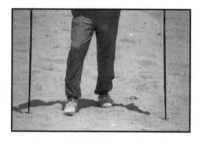

Photo 15-11. Using the poles for support at your sides, start by taking a few deep breaths to relax.

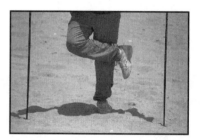

Photo 15-12. Cross one leg over your other knee, so your bent knee is at a 90-degree angle.

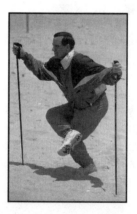

Photo 15-13. Keeping your back straight (it may lean slightly forward), bend the standing knee, allowing your body to become lower. As your derrière reaches the height of the standing knee, you'll feel the stretch in the bent knee hip joint.

Black Diamond Stretch

Let's give your hip joints a healthy stretch to really get them flexible. Along with your ability, this healthy stretch will help get you down the expert runs. Hold the stretch for each side for 15 seconds. Take the time to do it twice.

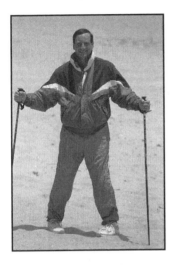

Photo 15-14. The key to this stretch is turning your toes in as you spread your legs slightly apart.

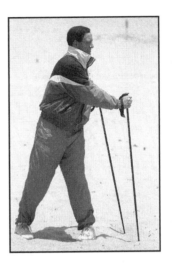

Photo 15-15. Rotate your body to one side. You'll feel the stretch in the opposite side hip joint.

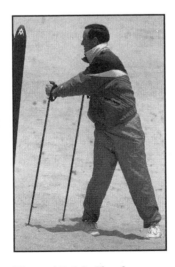

Photo 15-16. Slowly rotate to the other side.

205

Top of the Run Stretch

You're all stretched and ready to go. Unless you rode up in a gondola, you probably were sitting in the chairlift with your skis, bindings, and boots hanging down—a few pounds to say the least. Since they don't snow ski in Florida, I am assuming the temperature is somewhere below the freezing mark.

I'm sure you're nice and warm, but when you get off the chair, it may be a good idea for one more healthy stretch before your run. Actually, this stretch makes sense even if you did ride up in a gondola. All the muscles you'll be using get a last second wake-up call. Stretch just once and hold for 15 seconds. See you at the bottom!

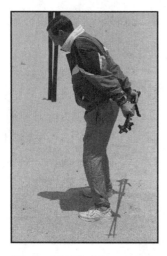

Photo 15-17. I haven't put my skis on yet, but I hold my poles behind my back.

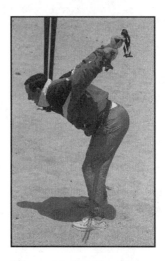

Photo 15-18. Keeping your back straight, lean forward slowly as you raise your arms. You'll feel the stretch in your torso, shoulders, and arms.

The Least You Need to Know

➤ Healthy stretching helps develop body awareness—something all great athletes have.

➤ Healthy stretching warms up the muscles for cold-weather performance.

➤ Your lower body acts like a shock absorber.

Part 5
Special Situations Require Special Stretches

Healthy stretching can be done during all the different stages of your life. I've included a pregnancy chapter along with stretching for children and seniors in this part of the book. If you want to get more out of life, don't let stiffness set in with inactivity. That's as true for children as it is for seniors.

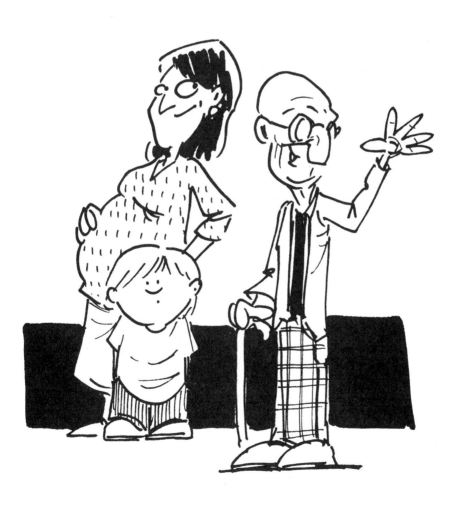

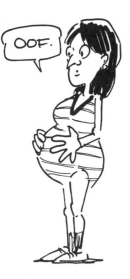

Chapter 16

Pregnancy Stretching: Expecting to Be Flexible

In This Chapter

➤ Healthy stretching during pregnancy will make you feel like leading a more active life

➤ Some healthy stretches to make mom merry

➤ Hold the stretch position for only 10 seconds

➤ Stretching with a partner or coach for confidence

Today's expectant mothers lead very active lifestyles, compared to years ago. Many women play tennis, golf, swim, and work out well into their pregnancies. Over the past few years, I've also noticed more and more pregnant women at my Boca Raton training center. Their desire to remain as flexible as possible, as their body undergoes changes, makes them dedicated clients.

Healthy Stretching During Pregnancy

Mr. Stretch Explains
Overstretching during pregnancy is possible because Relaxin, a hormone prevalent in the body during pregnancy to relax it for delivery, can also relax the connective tissue of the joints allowing an extension of their normal range of motion. Overextension can put damaging pressure on the nerves. Only stretch within your normal range of motion.

Mr. Stretch Explains
Holding for only 10 seconds for the healthy stretches in this chapter is like an insurance policy that protects your muscles from being stretched beyond their normal range of motion.

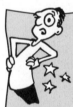

Chris's Concerns
It's very important to hold on to something, like a wall, for balance. Having confidence you won't fall allows you to get more from each healthy stretch. Sometimes it's a good idea, as in childbirth, to have a "coach" help you.

Healthy stretching is an ideal way for most women to stay flexible during the time leading up to the birth of their baby. Stretching's positive affect on the body's flexibility increases the desire to stay active. Feeling somewhat tired during pregnancy is normal, limiting the things you may want to do.

By healthy stretching, you can relieve some of your aches and pains and increase your desire to stay active, creating a positive frame of mind. Here's a list of some do's and don'ts for healthy stretching during pregnancy:

➤ DO hold the healthy stretches during pregnancy for only 10 seconds.

➤ DO check with your doctor for precautions and adaptations as you progress through the trimesters.

➤ DO healthy stretching to stay active and mobile.

➤ DO all healthy stretches slowly and gently and stay within a comfortable range of motion.

➤ DO have someone help you to boost your confidence.

➤ DON'T do any stretches you feel uncomfortable doing.

➤ DON'T *overstretch*.

Three "M" Stretches: Making Mom Merry

The first area we should give some healthy stretching to is your back. Carrying the weight of the ever-growing fetus has a tendency to make you lean forward, putting added pressure on the muscles of your back. These healthy stretches will help keep those muscles in the proper shape to help you support the load.

Back Bend-Over

Here's a healthy stretch for the lower back through to your shoulders. Sitting is something you're probably doing a lot more of as standing gets more tiring. I suggest doing this healthy stretch two times, *holding for only 10 seconds*.

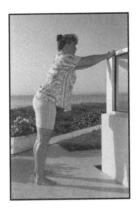

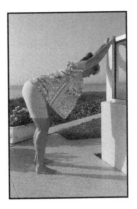

Photo 16-1. Stand like Jackie, with your hand against a wall or door that can't move. Spread your legs shoulder-width apart, knees slightly bent.

Photo 16-2. Bend over slowly, keeping your back straight, stretching your back muscles. Your head should not go past your hips. Hold for 10 seconds.

Standing Shoulder Twist

As your abdomen gets larger, your obliques, the muscles on the side of the stomach, get tighter. This healthy stretch will help achieve a proper length. Stretch twice for each side, holding for only 10 seconds.

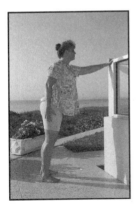

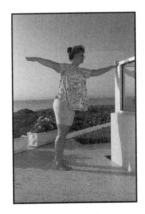

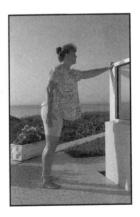

Photo 16-3. Stand facing the wall or a closed door that can't move. Place one hand on the wall.

Photo 16-4. Lift the other arm out from your side.

Photo 16-5. Slowly rotate to the side of the raised arm. The stretch position should form a straight line between both shoulders.

Crossover Stretch

One of the big problems my pregnant clients have is discomfort coming from the outside of their thighs up to the side of their abdomen. Muscle groups compensate for the shifting of weight and get tight. Stretch twice for each side, holding for 10 seconds.

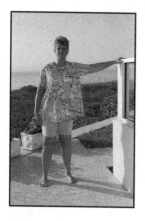

Photo 16-6. Stand sideways to the wall. Place your inner hand on the wall about shoulder height.

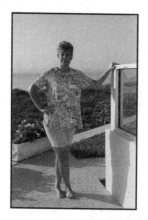

Photo 16-7. Cross the outside leg over the inside leg. Put your outside hand on your hip.

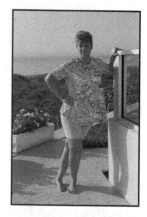

Photo 16-8. Lean your hips slowly to the wall. Bend your raised elbow to make it easier. You'll feel the stretch from the outside of your thigh up through the side of your abdomen.

Chris's Concerns
Dizziness or light-headedness can start as early as the fourth week, but usually starts in the second trimester. If at any time you get dizzy lying on your back, it's not a good idea to do these stretches. Since symptoms vary among individuals, I'm including them for your choice. These healthy stretches can also be done sitting.

Adjusting as You Adjust

As your body changes, you need to keep adjusting your muscles to reflect the changes. This next group of healthy stretches Jackie will be demonstrating deal with the support muscles that have to balance and carry the shifting additional weight. Do them very slowly and stay within your normal range of motion.

Knee-Neck Stretch

This healthy stretch will help your neck, shoulders, and leg muscles. Stretch each leg twice, holding for only 10 seconds.

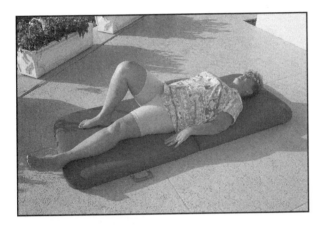

Photo 16-9. Lie down on your back and bend one knee.

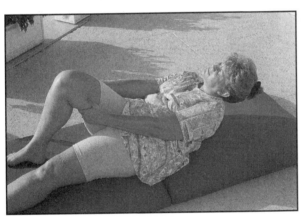

Photo 16-10. Reach your arms down slowly and grab the thigh of the bent leg. Notice Jackie is also leaning her head to the opposite shoulder.

Side Quad Stretch

The quads, the big muscles of the thigh, need some tender loving care. This healthy stretch should be done very slowly so you can feel the stretching of the quads and the abdominal muscles. Stretch twice for each leg, holding for only 10 seconds.

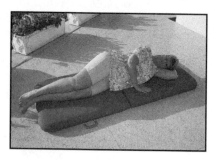

Photo 16-11. While lying on your side, put your lower hand under your head and place your upper hand on the mat.

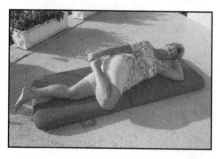

Photo 16-12. Bring your heel back as you reach down and hold your ankle.

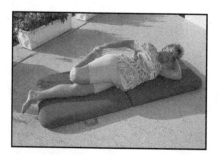

Photo 16-13. Stretch your heel slowly back and try to touch your derrière. Go only as far as is comfortable.

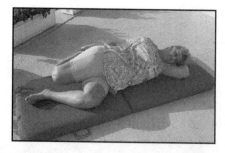

Photo 16-14. Slide your lower leg forward as you bend your knee for an additional stretch.

Two-Legged Pelvic Raise

This healthy stretch allows the stretching of several different muscle groups at the same time. You'll be stretching your quads and abdominals, while at the same time contracting your hamstrings and gluteus muscles to support the other muscles. This means you are making some opposing muscle groups work together. To stretch or lengthen the front muscles, you are contracting or working the muscles in the back of your thigh and in your buttocks to raise you up, providing support as you hold the stretch.

Stretch twice and hold for 10 seconds.

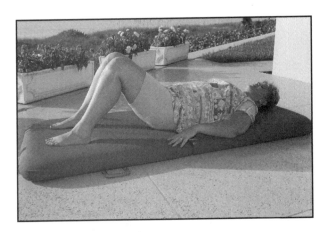

Photo 16-15. Lie on your back with your knees bent.

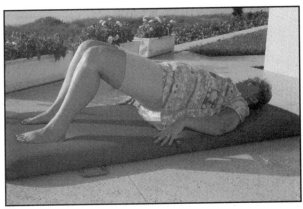

Photo 16-16. Raise your hips up so there is a tilted but straight line between your knees and shoulders.

Hamstring Stretch

Chris's Concerns
As you bring your leg up in the Hamstring stretch, do not bring your knee toward your chest. This would put pressure on your stomach. Stretch slowly and control your movements.

Your hamstring muscles, in the back of your thigh, will love this healthy stretch. You'll be able to walk around more comfortably if they're balanced to help the quads. Stretch each leg twice, holding for only 10 seconds.

Begin by lying on your back, knees bent, as shown in Photo 16-15.

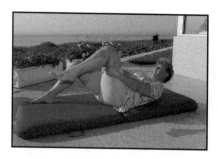

Photo 16-17. Reach with both hands and hold the back of your thigh, bringing it to a 90-degree angle.

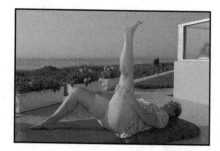

Photo 16-18. Raise your leg up, slowly straightening it, as high as you can comfortably raise it. You'll feel the stretch behind your knee in your hamstrings.

Let a Partner Help

You don't need a man to tell you this, but big changes are taking place as you get closer to the magic day. Getting lightheaded and feeling suddenly weak is not unusual. I really think it's a good idea to do these stretches with your partner or "coach" if you start to feel vulnerable. A coach will boost your confidence level as you communicate your needs and feelings.

Doug, Jackie's husband, is helping her do two of the healthy stretches. Notice how he provides support, guidance, and encouragement.

Partner Side Stretch

Your partner can help support and guide you through these side stretches. Communicate with each other and stretch slowly, maximizing the stretching benefits. You'll feel this stretch from mid-hip through your side up to your arm. Stretch each side twice, holding for 10 seconds.

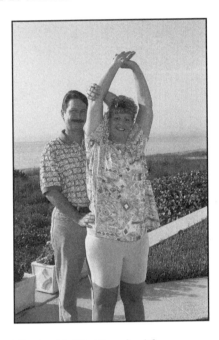

Photo 16-19. Stand with your arms above your head with your partner standing behind you. Doug's hands are on Jackie's hip and arm.

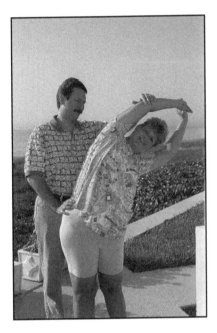

Photo 16-20. Jackie stretches slowly to her side. Doug is making sure she stretches only as far as she wants to.

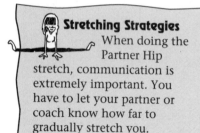

Partner Hip Stretch

This healthy stretch helps your hip joints. Your coach will help you push your knee up for the stretch, since reaching it might be difficult. Stretch each hip twice, holding for 10 seconds.

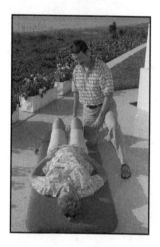

Photo 16-21. Lie down on your back with your knees bent. Your coach should be kneeling on the side that will be stretched.

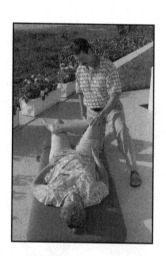

Photo 16-22. Cross one leg over the other. Your coach puts one hand on each knee.

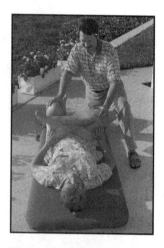

Photo 16-23. Your coach should stretch the bent knee toward your shoulder. You'll feel the stretch on the outside of your hips.

The Least You Need to Know

➤ You can healthy stretch away some of the aches and pains of pregnancy.

➤ It's important not to overstretch. Be sure to move into and out of each stretch slowly, maintaining normal breathing.

➤ Healthy stretching helps adjust muscle groups to the ever-changing requirements of pregnancy.

➤ Using a partner or coach can help provide stability, safety, and confidence.

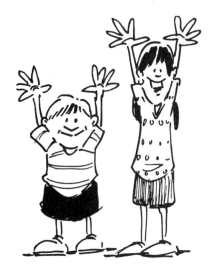

Chapter 17

Let's Stretch the Kids: Flexibility for Life

In This Chapter

➤ Children can be as tight as professional athletes

➤ Some kids suffer from growth-related diseases (as I did)

➤ Teenage sports injuries can be a result of juvenile flexibility problems

➤ Kids will have fun stretching, if you set a good example

This may really surprise you. The tightest, and I don't mean cheapest, athletes I see in my practice are tennis and soccer players and very active kids. You'd think with all the running around they do and their incredible energy, kids would be the ultimate example of perfect flexibility. Just the opposite can be true.

My Flexibility Problems as a Kid

Before looking into the future, let's discuss your children's present-day flexibility. Just like the rest of us, they may be flexible in certain areas while being tight in others. Just because your kids may do some incredibly flexible things doesn't mean their entire bodies are flexible. If your kids are flexible now, that doesn't mean that they'll remain flexible after puberty.

I'm a good example. When I was younger, I suffered from Osgood-Slaghter disease, a growth-related disease affecting the patella tendon. It connects the quad muscle to a growth plate below the kneecap. As I grew, the tendon had a tendency to pull away from the growth plate and calcium formed, creating bumps. It was very painful. Doctors used to treat it by putting kids in casts. Today, it's treated by telling kids to rest when the pain becomes severe.

Mr. Stretch Explains
Kids go through quick growth spurts, sometimes growing three to six inches taller in one year. The rapid growth can create tightness. Healthy stretching educates muscles to adapt to the lengths the body needs in order to rotate properly.

Now I realize that inflexibility in the quad and hip flexor muscles contributes to this and other growth-related conditions. Tight hamstrings and inner thigh muscles can also put pressure on the quad muscles, creating a problem. If you wonder why I'm suggesting you take your children's flexibility seriously, now you know. Maybe we should consider some conditions flexibility problems rather than growth problems.

Be a Flexibility-Conscious Parent

Setting a good example is one of the best ways to instill the importance of flexibility in your kids. I find that kids who stretch with their parents enjoy and value stretching later in life. You can use this time as quality playtime. If kids think it's important and fun, they'll do some healthy stretching. *I find a similar situation with some of my professional athletic clients.*

Mr. Stretch Explains
I find a similar situation with some of my professional athletic clients. When I start working with a new professional client, they very often don't understand how healthy stretching improves their performance levels, until I show them and they realize their untapped potential.

Have your kids ever told you they don't like a particular sport? Very often it's because their bodies can't adapt to the sport. I see it a lot in junior golf and tennis. Kids get discouraged because their bodies won't let them develop the techniques they're being taught.

Some of the injuries that happen to kids playing high school baseball, for example, are a result of inflexibility problems from when they played Little League baseball. With so many kids taking up golf, because of Tiger Woods, the same could happen—unless their bodies are prepared to play. Healthy stretching will help avoid these problems, but you have to help too by setting a good example and making it fun.

Children Are Sitters Too!

Computers, video games, and television take up lots of a kid's time. You may think your kids are always active—but are they really? Just for fun, keep a log on the amount of time you see them sitting. I'm not being critical of the amount of time they sit, just trying to make you aware of some flexibility problems healthy stretching can correct. If, on the other hand, you have a child who is lethargic, meaning a child who doesn't like to do very much except lay around the house, remember that lethargy promotes lethargy. If we can devise a way to make healthy stretching fun, you'll have a child who feels better and wants to increase his or her activities.

How to Start—Become Mr. Stretch's Assistant Coach

With kids who love sports and watch a lot of it on television, have them stretch while watching. Use some of the healthy stretches in this chapter and tell them it's time they had a pre-game stretching routine, just like the players.

If you take them to college or pro sporting events, go a little early to watch the athletes prepare for the game. The teams usually come on the field or court to stretch about an hour before the scheduled start. Let their heroes set a good example.

If your child sits a lot, you can use some of the healthy stretches in Chapter 8. Make them fun. I know they'll definitely enjoy the Programmer stretches.

The best way to begin is to take Chapter 1's flexibility test together. Compare your flexibility in different areas. It's a positive activity to do with your children and gives you a pretty good idea of whether any flexibility problems exist or are starting—for all of you.

Want one final good argument to start your kids on a lifetime of flexibility? My senior clients tell me that if they knew they were going to live as long as they have, they would have taken better care of themselves. Insurance companies' actuary tables that deal with life span prove our lives are getting longer.

Make sure your kids don't have to experience some of the painful problems and injuries a lot of senior citizens cope with. Help them learn about the benefits of flexibility now.

Fun Favorites

When you were younger, didn't you enjoy walking on the edge of the curb to see if you could keep your balance? That's not all bad—unless it's a busy street and traffic is coming. You were teaching yourself body awareness.

These healthy stretches are great for kids to do with each other. The demonstrators are Adam and Jordan and their Mom, Ellen. Adam is an active soccer player, Mom's an "A" list tennis player, and Jordan, well, he's very active and learns fast. They are an active family; everyone water skis but, like all kids, Adam and Jordan are not as flexible as they could be. These healthy stretches will help.

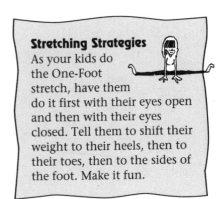

Stretching Strategies
As your kids do the One-Foot stretch, have them do it first with their eyes open and then with their eyes closed. Tell them to shift their weight to their heels, then to their toes, then to the sides of the foot. Make it fun.

One-Foot Stretch

Kids love to do this because they want to see "How long can I stand on one foot?" It also teaches body awareness, since they have to make adjustments to stay balanced. Holding time is not important, since they'll compete to see who can do it longer. Have them balance on both legs.

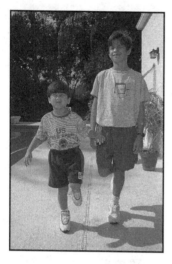

Photo 17-1. Jordan and Adam stand on one leg.

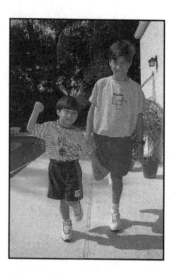

Photo 17-2. Jordan is making some balance adjustments and developing his body awareness.

Feeling Taller

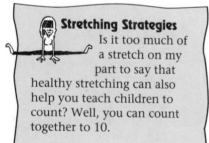

Stretching Strategies
Is it too much of a stretch on my part to say that healthy stretching can also help you teach children to count? Well, you can count together to 10.

All kids want to pretend they're taller. You can play along and help them feel taller with this healthy stretch. Maybe even make a mark against a wall and have them do the Hands Above the Head stretch once a week to see if they can reach higher. No jumping allowed. Have them hold it for five to 10 seconds.

Hands Above the Head Stretch

Play a game with your children. Have them imitate you as you reach as high as you can.

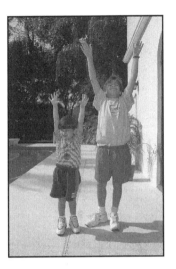

Photo 17-3. How high can you reach, kids?

Soccer Stretch

Have your children reach back and hold a foot. This is a stretch for the quads, the muscles in front of the thigh. The more advanced stretches have you pull the leg back. For children, just have them hold their foot and try to touch their bottom with it.

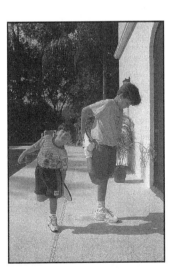

Photo 17-4. Can you touch your foot to your bottom?

Side Stretch

This is a great exercise to help your children with. You can communicate with each other as you help them get into position. The key is to let them feel they're in control. Stretch each side a couple of times holding for five to 10 seconds.

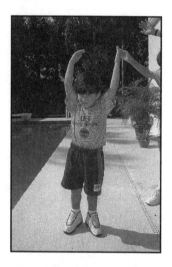

Photo 17-5. Ask your child to reach up high like Jordan.

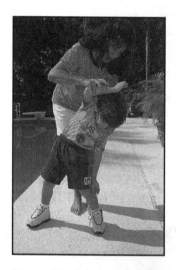

Photo 17-6. Stand behind and start helping your child lean to one side. Remind him or her to take some deep breaths while stretching.

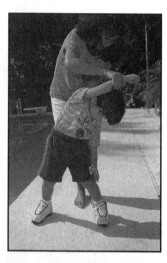

Photo 17-7. Try to help your child go a little further each time.

Cannon Ball

This is a fun stretch to help out the spine. Kids love to do this one. Start by having them lay on the ground and then rock back and forth a few times.

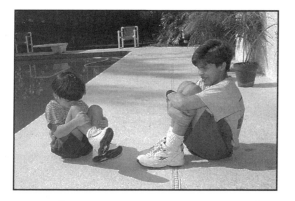

Photo 17-8. Have your children sit and bring their knees up to their chest.

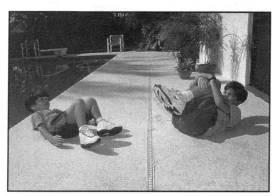

Photo 17-9. Have your children rock back. (Jordan has lost his grip. If this happens, they'll get it right next time.)

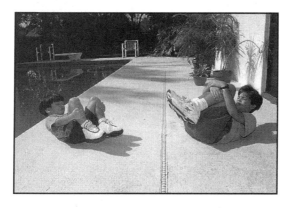

Photo 17-10. Adam and Jordan are rocking back as far as they can go. Have your child rock back and forth, massaging the spine.

Back Leaner

This healthy stretch is a fun way to work on the quads and front muscles of the abdomen. Have them do it slowly (lots of luck) and try to hold the leaning position for five to 10 seconds. Repeat one more time.

Photo 17-11. Have your children begin on their knees. Feet should be behind them and their posture should be straight.

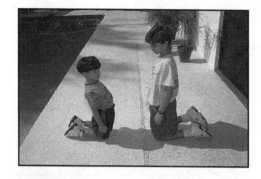

Photo 17-12. Tell your children to slowly lean back.

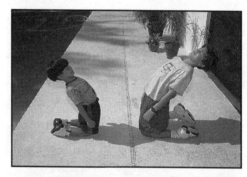

Photo 17-13. Have them go back as far as they can comfortably go. They should not feel this stretch in their backs, only in their quads and muscles in the front of the abdomen.

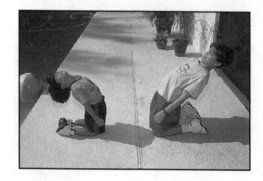

Hamstring Stretch

In Photo 17-14, Adam is demonstrating what you're likely to see if children have tight hamstrings. They can't stretch their feet out and sit straight. Older children can do this stretch by themselves. You'll want to help the younger ones. Stretch each leg slowly for five to 10 seconds and repeat twice.

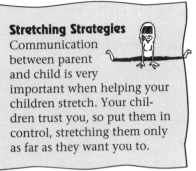

Stretching Strategies
Communication between parent and child is very important when helping your children stretch. Your children trust you, so put them in control, stretching them only as far as they want you to.

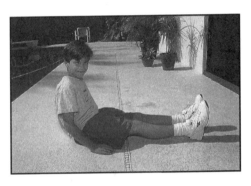

Photo 17-14. Start by having your child sit up as straight as possible with legs stretched out in front.

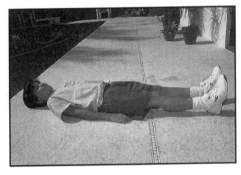

Photo 17-15. The child should slowly lean back until he or she is flat on the ground.

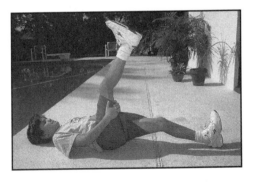

Photo 17-16. Adam is raising one leg and stretching it up with his hands wrapped behind his knee.

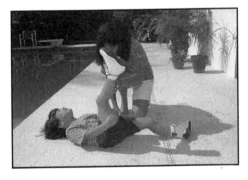

Photo 17-17. Help your younger children raise their leg as Ellen is doing with Jordan.

Campfire Sitting Stretch

Stretching Strategies
Make sure your kids are doing the stretches correctly. I work with camps where everybody does the stretch together. They don't go on to the next one until everyone does it correctly.

Some kids can't sit campfire style because their hips are too tight. This is a good stretch for them and fun to do. Have them hold this position for 15 seconds.

Photo 17-18. Ask your kids to sit and cross their legs. Having the kids sit straighter helps this healthy stretch.

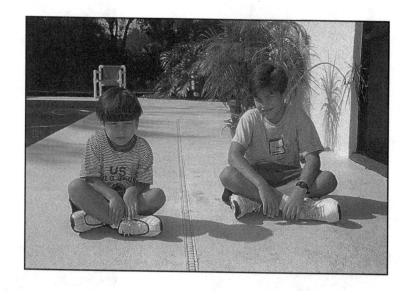

Swordsmen Lunge

Your kids can pretend to be swordsmen. Help your kids make this into a game. This healthy stretch is for the quads and hamstrings. Do each leg twice, holding for 10 seconds.

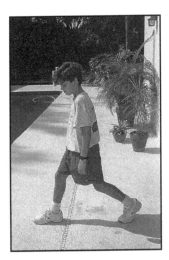

Photo 17-19. To start, have your child put one foot back a few feet and stand up straight.

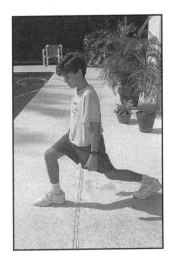

Photo 17-20. Adam is stretching his hips forward while keeping his torso straight. Be sure the front knee doesn't go past the front foot. The stretch should be felt in the quad of his front leg and the hamstring of the back leg.

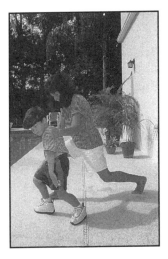

Photo 17-21. Mom is helping young Jordan get into the proper stretching position.

Neck Stretches

This is a great way for both kids and parents to stretch away some tension together. It's fun to do in front of a mirror, slowly. The kids get to watch as their parent's head goes one way while theirs goes the other way. Repeat at least twice slowly and hold for 15 seconds. You deserve this relaxing moment.

Photo 17-22. After starting with your heads straight, you slowly stretch to one side while your child stretches to the other. Reverse direction slowly.

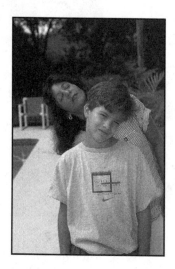

The Least You Need to Know

➤ Children are not always as flexible as you think.

➤ Family stretching is quality time spent with your kids.

➤ Healthy stretching provides for a flexible life.

➤ Be sure your children stretch correctly.

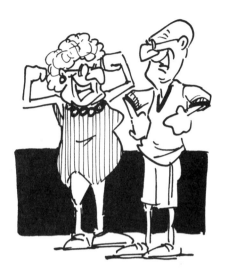

Chapter 18

Senior Flexibility: Healthy Stretching for an Active Lifestyle

In This Chapter

➤ Healthy stretching has helped many seniors become more active

➤ Even if you've sought other remedies, healthy stretching can help you get rid of aches and pains

➤ Healthy stretching allows your joints to rotate more freely

➤ Keeping your hip joint stretched can help eliminate the need for a hip replacement

I enjoy working with seniors. Many have searched all over trying to eliminate pain and inflexibility. Carolyn, our 86-and-a-half-year-old demonstrator for this chapter, is a good example. The pain from a broken back in an auto accident 10 years ago made her seek the help of pain management specialists, chiropractors, and several massage therapists along with doctors. I'm not criticizing any of those individuals or professions, just using them as an example to illustrate how desperately she wanted to feel well again.

How Healthy Stretching Helped Carolyn

Mr. Stretch Explains
A *locked hip* means the muscle groups that connect to the hip have shortened to the point that they severely restrict hip rotation. It's painful and makes other muscles groups pick up the load, sometimes injuring them as well. Locked hips, for example, can cause inner-thigh strains.

Carolyn read a story about my Chris Verna Training Center in the *Palm Beach Post* and called requesting an appointment. After explaining the type of pain and discomfort symptoms she was feeling, I satisfied myself that her medical history would allow some stretching. Within 10 minutes of being on my table, the source of her pain, a *locked hip*, was corrected.

Carolyn is now the active woman she once was. You'd be amazed at the schedule she keeps. She loves helping people and volunteers for many endeavors. I'm really happy that healthy stretching has helped her regain and maintain her flexibility. By the way, Carolyn is now more flexible than some kids when they first come to see me.

*Photo 18-1.
Carolyn and
Mr. Stretch.*

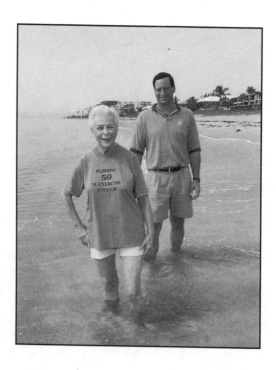

Mr. Stretch, Can Healthy Stretching Help Me Too?

Most likely the answer is yes. Most of the stiffness and discomfort you are experiencing is caused by muscles that have become shortened and tight. Healthy stretching keeps your muscles more elastic and ready to respond to your needs. Just like Carolyn, some of your problems could have set in years ago. Here are some suggestions:

➤ Start by taking the flexibility self-test in Chapter 1. Do it slowly to pinpoint your flexibility problems in specific body areas.

➤ Use Chapter 2 to find any other clues that may be causing your restricted flexibility.

➤ Start by doing the senior healthy stretches in this chapter. Carolyn is doing them so you can feel secure that you can do them too!

➤ If the healthy stretches are making you feel better, which they should, consider doing the stretches in Part 6. They're arranged by specific body areas.

➤ If you do nothing else, try to move as much as possible. Make yourself stay active and use your muscles.

Chris's Concerns

If you have been inactive because of medical situations, I suggest discussing healthy stretching with your doctor. For most seniors, healthy stretching can help you feel better, increasing your desire to do more activities.

Senior Savvy Stretches

My senior clients start with some easy stretches to loosen up their torso and shoulder muscles first. At my suggestion, Carolyn does these stretches twice a day.

When you stretch, take some deep breaths and relax. As your personal stretching coach, I want you to enjoy feeling looser again. Do each stretch slowly and gently. Each time you do the stretch, try to go just a little bit farther, gradually increasing your range of motion. I want to be totally honest with you: Carolyn is now very flexible, so we had her limit the hold positions she's demonstrating to accommodate the range of motion of less flexible seniors.

Stretching Strategies

Sometimes it's a good idea to stretch with a partner or friend. You both can communicate how you're feeling and make sure the other is doing the stretch correctly. Never rush. Healthy stretching should be done very slowly, so you can feel the muscles lengthen.

Overhead Side Stretch

> **Stretching Strategies**
> Be sure your feet are more than shoulder-width apart as you do the Overhead Side stretch. The wider stance will give you a very solid base so you won't feel like you're falling over. It also positions the muscles properly for stretching.

This healthy stretch will gently stretch the muscles from the top of your hip through your arm. Slowly and gently is the best way to stretch so that you can feel how far you should go. Stretch each side three times, holding for 15 seconds.

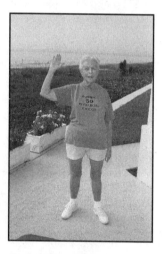

Photo 18-2. Stand straight with your feet spread more than shoulder-width apart. One arm should be at your side while the other is bent forming about a 90-degree angle.

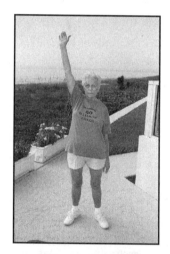

Photo 18-3. Straighten your arm by lifting it up. Doing it slowly will allow you to feel a slight stretching in the arm.

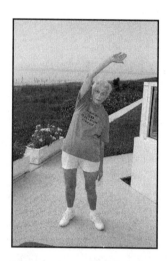

Photo 18-4. Slowly stretch to the side as far as you can comfortably go. You'll feel the stretch starting above your hip.

Standing Shoulder Twist

If you want to increase your rotational flexibility, this healthy stretch can help. Once again, do it slowly so that you can feel the muscles of your torso stretch. Stretch each side three times, holding for 15 seconds.

You may want to do these rotational twist stretches in front of a mirror. Observe whether one side is not able to turn back as much as the other. If that's the case, stretch the more flexible side twice and the stiffer side three times to balance the muscle groups.

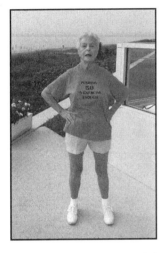

Photo 18-5. Stand straight with your hands on your hips. Spread your feet slightly wider than shoulder-width apart.

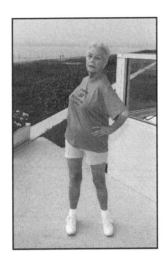

Photo 18-6. Stretch your shoulders back and to one side. You'll feel a twisting stretch across your lower torso.

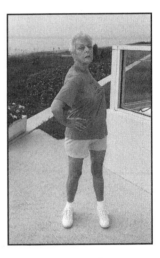

Photo 18-7. Feel your lower body rotate and stretch from one side to the other.

235

Cross-Body Arm Stretch

This healthy stretch helps your shoulders, arms, and the area between the shoulder blades of your mid-back. Once again, a nice slow stretch will help you feel better. Stretch each side three times, holding for 15 seconds.

The goal of the Cross-Body Arm stretch is to eventually bring your arm as close to your chest as possible. Healthy stretching allows that to happen gradually without damaging the muscle. Try to slowly stretch a little bit farther each time.

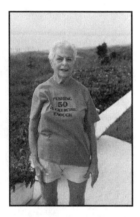

Photo 18-8. Stand straight and take a nice relaxing deep breath.

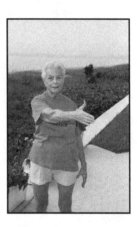

Photo 18-9. Start bringing your arm across your body, but do not twist your shoulders. Still face straight ahead.

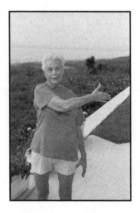

Photo 18-10. This may be as far as you can comfortably go, as you bring your arm across your body.

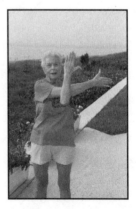

Photo 18-11. Take your other arm and wrap it outside your across-the-body arm. Slowly and gently stretch it toward your chest. You'll feel the stretch in your shoulder and shoulder blades.

The "Flexibility Five" Stretches

The next five healthy stretches are designed to be done on the ground. A mat or thick towel would be ideal to offer some comfortable support. You'll be able to comfortably stretch the muscles groups that may be responsible for causing your discomfort.

Hips, shoulders, and upper backs will get some tender loving care as you stretch them to their proper lengths. Stretch slowly; feeling the muscles lengthen is key. As you stretch you'll also be building up your confidence level. Once your flexibility returns, some aches and pains will disappear and you'll feel more like participating in all sorts of activities.

En Garde

The next two healthy stretches are lunges. That doesn't mean you have to quickly plant your front foot forward or to the side. But it's similar to a swordsman position in a duel. If I had been the stretching coach for King Arthur and his Knights of the Round Table, Camelot might have been known more for lower body flexibility then for chivalry.

Now, it's time to healthy stretch your legs. We'll begin by stretching your quads and hamstrings—the big muscles in your thigh—and your lower leg muscles in the calves. Stretch slowly is the key phrase, as each leg is stretched two or three times. Hold for 15 seconds.

Chris's Concerns
You should not feel any stretching in your lower back as you do the En Garde stretch. Be sure to re-check your position with the demonstration—you may be leaning too far forward.

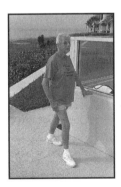

Photo 18-12. Place one foot behind the other with your hands to your sides. Balance yourself by placing one hand on a wall.

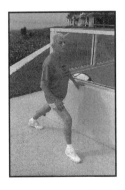

Photo 18-13. Move your back foot as far back as it will comfortably go.

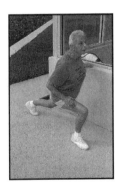

Photo 18-14. Lean your hips forward as you bend your knee. Notice how Carolyn does not lean her upper body forward. She's keeping her shoulders above her hips.

237

Side Lunge

Let's do one more lunge stretch to help the inner-thigh muscles. Slowly stretch each leg two or three times and hold for 15 seconds.

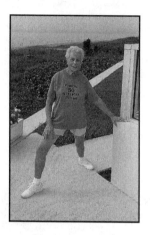

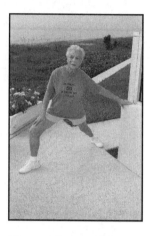

Photo 18-15. Have something sturdy close by to hold onto for balance support. Take a step to the side keeping your back foot facing forward and the foot you stepped with pointing sideways.

Photo 18-16. Slide your back foot back as you lean your hips forward.

Senior Hamstring Stretch

Stretching Strategies

If you prefer not to try all the positions in the Senior Hamstring stretch, that's okay. Stretch only as far as you want and hold that position for 15 seconds. Every little bit of stretching helps. The more flexible you feel, the farther you may want to stretch.

The hamstrings help you balance as you walk. If you've been doing a lot of sitting, these big muscles really need some healthy stretching. This stretch will help improve your hip rotation. Slowly stretch each leg twice and hold for 10 seconds.

While in the same position as Photo 18-18, you can also stretch your shoulders by moving your knee back down. This puts stretching tension on the shoulders and gives them a great healthy stretch.

238

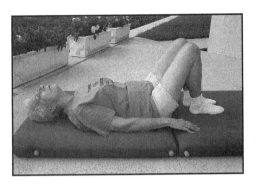

Photo 18-17. Lie on your back, knees bent, and hands to your sides.

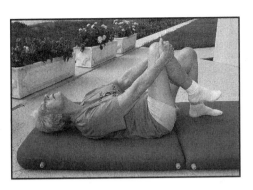

Photo 18-18. Reach and hold one leg with both hands around your knee and stretch it slowly toward your chest.

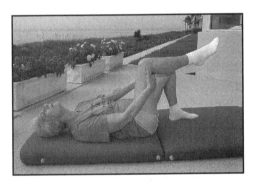

Photo 18-19. Move your hands under your knee so they hold your thigh. Slowly raise the foot of the bent knee so that it's parallel with the ground.

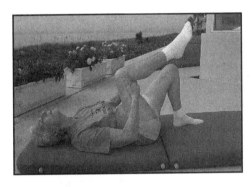

Photo 18-20. Stretch your knee farther toward your chest.

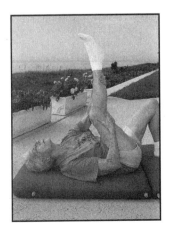

Photo 18-21. Reach one hand up toward your ankle, while the other hand stays behind your knee. Slowly stretch as you straighten your leg. You'll feel this extended stretch behind your knee.

Senior Modified Pretzel

This is a great healthy stretch to help prevent hip replacement surgery. It's a gentle exercise that uses the leverage of your knee to help stretch your hip joint. Stretch each leg twice, holding for 15 seconds.

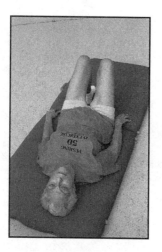

Photo 18-22. Lie on your back with knees bent, hands at your sides.

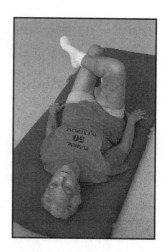

Photo 18-23. Cross one leg so that you rest your ankle just below your other knee.

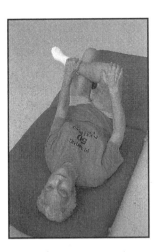

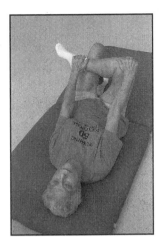

Photo 18-24. Place one hand on the knee and your other hand on your ankle.

Photo 18-25. Push gently but firmly on your knee to stretch the hip joint.

Senior Side-Quad Stretch

By lying down, you won't have to worry about losing your balance as you stretch your quads. Stretch slowly and feel the big muscles in the front of your thigh stretch. I suggest doing each leg at least twice, holding for 10 seconds.

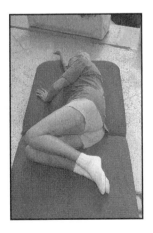

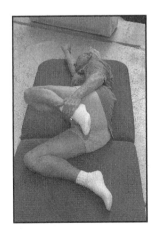

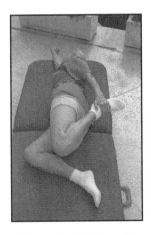

Photo 18-26. Lie on your side with both knees bent.

Photo 18-27. Reach down and hold your top ankle.

Photo 18-28. Stretch your leg back but do not move the lower leg. You'll feel the stretch in the front of your thigh.

241

The Least You Need to Know

➤ Healthy stretching can be the start of your fitness program.

➤ Healthy stretching may help you feel better, even if you've searched for a cure for years.

➤ Healthy stretching allows your joints to rotate freely.

➤ Keeping your hip joint stretched can help prevent hip replacement surgery.

➤ Stretching slowly helps build confidence.

Part 6

Mr. Stretch's Program for Improving the Quality of Your Life With Stretching

From your toes to your neck, (remember I believe that energy flows upward), you'll find some healthy stretches to help get your body rotating freely again.

If you've come to this part of the Guide as a result of finding a problem in the Chapter 1 flexibility self-test, you'll find it's divided into various chapters featuring stretches for the various regions of your body.

Remember, with healthy stretching, the more flexible you become, the less you have to do. Your new body awareness will help you detect when a problem may be starting. This section of the book will help you correct it.

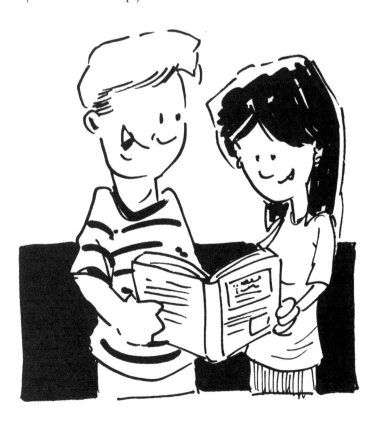

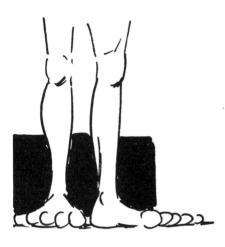

Chapter 19

Healthy Stretching Your Feet, Ankles, and Calves

In This Chapter

➤ For lower leg flexibility problems, try some healthy stretches in this chapter

➤ Healthy stretches for the feet, ankles, and calves to improve the flexibility of your lower leg

Lower leg inflexibility is usually a result of stiffness in your feet, ankles, or calves (the shaded areas in Figure 19-1). To correct the problem, I suggest mixing together healthy stretches for all three areas. As you stretch, you'll be able to determine where the problem is coming from.

*Figure 19-1. Feet,
ankles, and calves.*

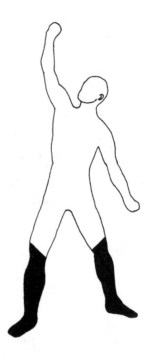

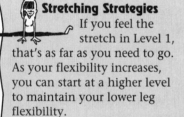

Stretching Strategies
If you feel the stretch in Level 1, that's as far as you need to go. As your flexibility increases, you can start at a higher level to maintain your lower leg flexibility.

Standing Calf Stretch

This healthy stretch works on both sides of the calves. It's a Level 1 stretch, which means it begins the stretching of the area. Other levels will provide help, once the calf is flexible enough to take advantage of the advanced stretch. You'll feel the stretch from the heel to the knee. Alternate legs as you slowly stretch each leg twice, holding for 15 seconds in both stretch positions.

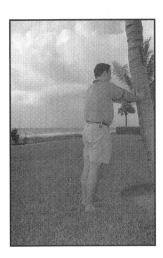

Photo 19-1. Stand with your hands resting on a tree or wall.

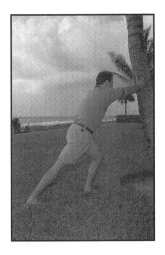

Photo 19-2. Step back with one leg and lean your body forward. Don't let your knee go farther forward than your foot.

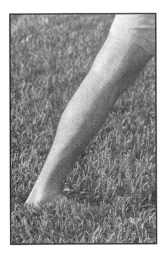

Photo 19-3. Your leg should be straight with your heel on the ground. You'll feel the stretch in the back of your calf. Hold for 15 seconds.

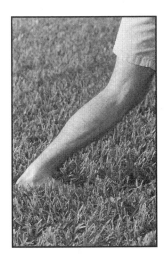

Photo 19-4. Bend your knee forward to stretch the muscle in front of your calves. Heel still is on the ground. Hold for 15 seconds.

247

Level 2 Standing Heel and Calf Stretch

I'm using my sea wall to do this, but you can use the lowest step on your staircase or walkway. Stand straight as you stretch slowly and you'll feel your ankle and calves stretching. Alternate feet and stretch twice, holding for 15 seconds.

Photo 19-5. Stand backwards and slide one foot back so that your heel is not on the step.

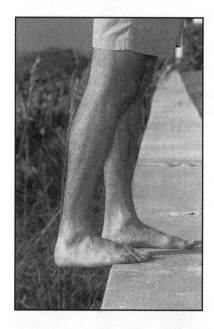

Photo 19-6. Stretch your ankle slowly down and feel your calf stretching from your ankle to the back of your knee.

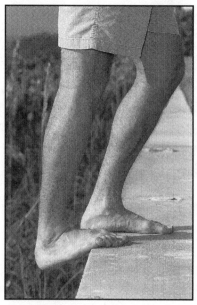

Level 3 Heel and Calf Stretch

If you're flexible in the lower leg, this Level 3 stretch will maintain your flexibility. It's an intensive stretch that you'll feel more in the back of your knee. You can use a wall or doorway. Hold onto the wall or door molding for balance. Alternate and stretch each leg twice, holding for 15 seconds.

Stretching Strategies
This Level 3 healthy stretch is for someone who really needs flexible ankles, like a runner, hiker, or climber. I suggest doing Level 2 first before doing this intensive stretch. It's especially effective if you don't lean forward as you stretch.

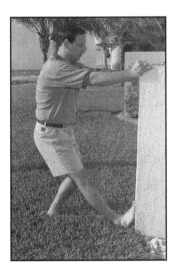

Photo 19-7. Put your heel close to a wall. You may have to lower your derrière to get your heel as close as possible.

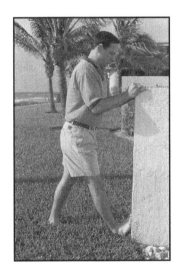

Photo 19-8. Once your heel is in place, stretch your knee closer to the wall by bringing your hips closer to the wall.

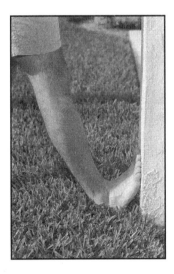

Photo 19-9. A close-up view of the hold position.

Shin Splint Stretch

This is an excellent stretch for runners because you have to pick up your toes to make a stride. Scuffing along is a symptom you need this healthy stretch. It's also good for hikers, climbers, and tennis players.

So let's stretch the front of your leg, the shin. You can regulate the amount of stretch by how far back you lower your hips. Go only as far as is comfortable. The amount of stretch and your flexibility can be increased with each repetition. Stretch each leg twice, holding for 15 seconds.

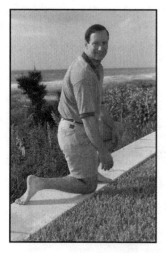

Photo 19-10. Kneel down on one knee, with your foot out behind you. Rest the top of your toes on the ground, keeping a straight upper body.

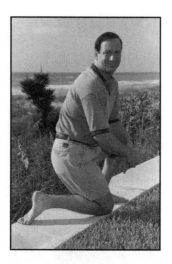

Photo 19-11. Start to sit back on your foot. If you feel the stretch early on, hold in that position for 15 seconds.

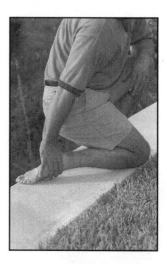

Photo 19-12. For a more intensive stretch, reach back to hold your heel as you sit all the way back.

Outside of Ankle Stretch

This is similar to the Shin Splint stretch, but it also healthy stretches the ankle. If you've ever sprained your ankle or had problems with your shins, it's a great way to help regain your flexibility. The amount of stretch can be regulated by how far back you sit. Each leg should be stretched twice, holding for 15 seconds.

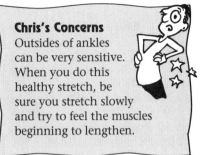

Chris's Concerns
Outsides of ankles can be very sensitive. When you do this healthy stretch, be sure you stretch slowly and try to feel the muscles beginning to lengthen.

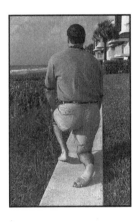

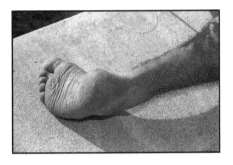

Photo 19-14. This is how your foot should be turned in.

Photo 19-13. Kneel on one knee, keeping your upper body straight with your leg behind you. Turn your foot in.

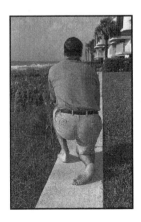

Photo 19-15. Start to sit back on your foot. If you feel the stretch early on, hold in that position for 15 seconds.

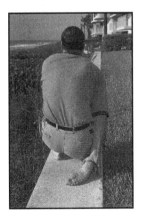

Photo 19-16. For a more intensive stretch, reach back, holding your heel as you sit all the way back.

251

The Toe and Foot stretch should be done to prevent shortening of the tendons due to age. The tendons get shorter from fatigue and lack of use. Healthy stretching can prevent these problems from occurring.

Toe and Foot Stretch

This healthy stretch is for the muscles of your toes. You'll feel it on the top of your foot, especially if you tend to keep your toes up when you stand. The best time to do this is every morning before you put your shoes on and every night after you take your shoes off. If you're a "stander," do these healthy stretches several times during the day. Stretch each foot twice, holding for 15 seconds.

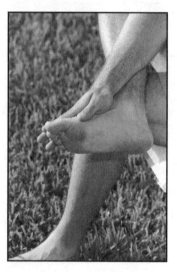

Photo 19-17. Cross one foot over your knee. Place your hand on top of your foot so each finger is in line with a toe.

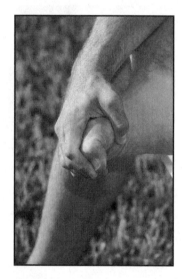

Photo 19-18. Curl your toes down, stretching them, using your hand. You'll feel the tendons on the top of your foot stretch. Hold for 15 seconds.

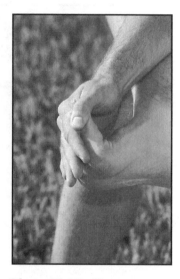

Photo 19-19. Now put your fingers on the bottom of your foot and pull your fingers up so you stretch the toes in the opposite direction. Hold for 15 seconds.

Ankle Rotation

Another good healthy stretch to do while you're sitting is the Ankle Rotation. It's a great way to condition your ankles to the rotation that's required to help you walk or move quickly. If you have a tendency to stumble, tight ankles may be part of the problem.

As you slowly rotate the ankle around, a body awareness of your ankles rotating develops while you are stretching them. Stretch both ankles as you rotate them 360 degrees.

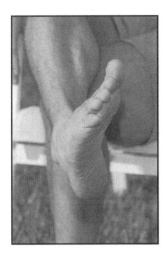

Photo 19-20. Stretch your ankle to one side.

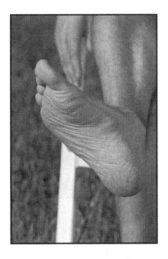

Photo 19-21. Stretch your ankle to the other side.

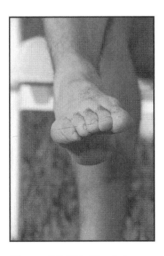

Photo 19-22. Stretch your ankle down.

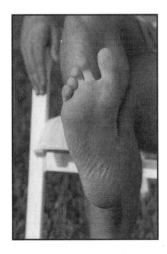

Photo 19-23. Stretch your ankle up.

253

The Least You Need to Know

➤ Healthy stretching helps develop body awareness, allowing quicker reaction to changing terrain and preventing stumbles and falls.

➤ Healthy stretching helps prevent the natural shortening of your toe and foot tendons due to aging.

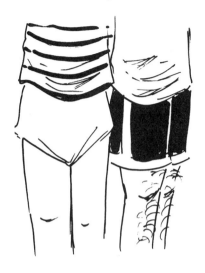

Chapter 20

Healthy Stretching Your Knees, Hips, and Hamstrings

In This Chapter

➤ Healthy stretches for flexibility problems in your knees, hips, or hamstrings

➤ Knee inflexibility may be caused by a hip flexibility problem

---

Body flexibility is based on various muscle groups working together. As an example, in opposing muscle groups, one group lengthens while the other contracts. In certain situations—the knees, for example—the muscle groups of the hip are also connected below the knee. That means a knee problem may be a result of a hip flexibility problem. The knees, hips, and hamstrings, as shaded in Figure 20-1, all depend on each other.

I believe it's important to stretch several muscle groups to be sure the real problem has been discovered and corrected. The Chapter 1 flexibility self-test may have discovered some problems and suggested you consult this chapter. It's usually best to do these healthy stretches in order. As soon as your flexibility problem improves, you can eliminate or vary the stretches. Once a muscle is stretched to its proper length, you don't need to stretch it any further. Maintaining the muscle's flexibility is the goal.

Figure 20-1. Knees, hips, and hamstrings.

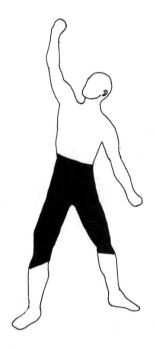

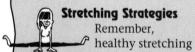

Stretching Strategies
Remember, healthy stretching doesn't mean that you rush and force the joints to move. Even a small improvement in your range of motion is a step forward.

Pretzel Stretch

This series of healthy stretches will help you gain flexibility in your tight hips. I'll demonstrate some different levels. Begin with Level 1 and proceed to higher levels as your flexibility allows.

Modified Pretzel Stretch

If your hips are especially tight, or if you're a senior citizen, try starting with this modified healthy stretch. Alternate and slowly stretch each side twice, holding for 15 seconds. You should feel the stretch in the base of your derrière or the back of your hip to the outside of the leg being stretched.

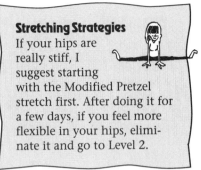

Stretching Strategies

If your hips are really stiff, I suggest starting with the Modified Pretzel stretch first. After doing it for a few days, if you feel more flexible in your hips, eliminate it and go to Level 2.

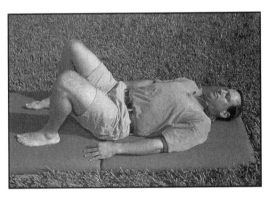

Photo 20-1. As you lie flat on your back, bend your knees.

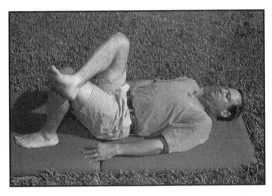

Photo 20-2. Cross one leg, placing your heel over the knee of the opposite leg.

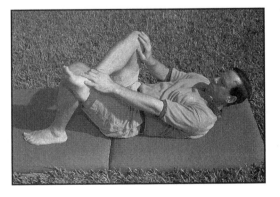

Photo 20-3. Place one hand on your knee, the other hand on your ankle.

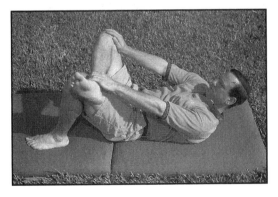

Photo 20-4. Push gently but firmly on the knee, trying to get it parallel to your hips.

Full Pretzel Stretch

Everyone needs to stretch out their hips. This Full Pretzel stretch will help correct most hip flexibility problems. Do it slowly and feel your muscles stretch. Try to stretch a little farther each time until you can establish a full range of motion. Alternate legs and stretch twice, holding for 15 seconds.

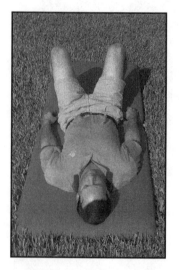

Photo 20-5. Start by lying on your back, hands to your side, and knees bent.

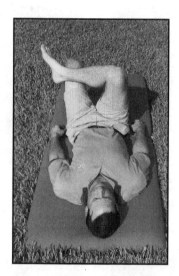

Photo 20-6. Cross one leg so the heel rests on the opposite knee.

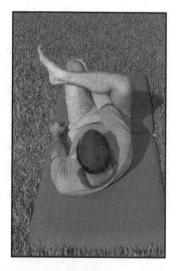

Photo 20-7. Reach forward, with your hand from the same side as the crossed leg, through the gap in your legs and hold your bent knee. Your hips and torso will come toward each other.

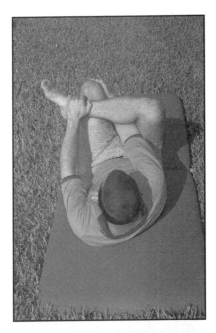

Photo 20-8. Place your other hand on the crossed-over ankle for leverage. This is a Level 2 flexibility position.

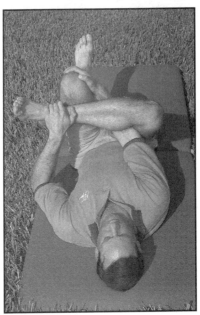

Photo 20-9. Slowly lie flat on the ground to increase the stretch. This is a Level 3 flexibility position.

Seated Hip Stretch

This healthy stretch can be conveniently done at various times during the day while sitting. It will improve your hip rotation, which also corrects the Waddling Duck image you may have discovered in Chapter 1's flexibility self-test. Stretch slowly, trying to bring your crossed-over leg as flat as possible. Alternate and stretch each leg twice, holding for 15 seconds. See, you can do this anywhere.

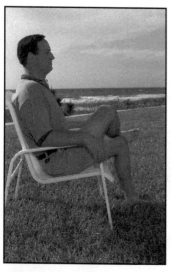

Photo 20-10. Sit with your back straight up against the chair. Cross one leg over the knee of the other. Remember, your inflexibility is determined by how high your knee is popped up.

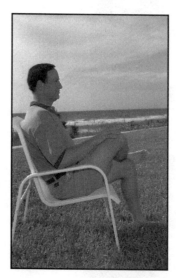

Photo 20-11. Put your hand on your knee. Since I'm stretching my right hip, I'm placing my right hand on the crossed-over knee.

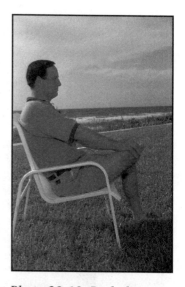

Photo 20-12. Push down on the knee to stretch it even with your other knee. You'll feel the stretch in your hip joint or other surrounding areas that may also be tight. This is a Level 1 flexibility position.

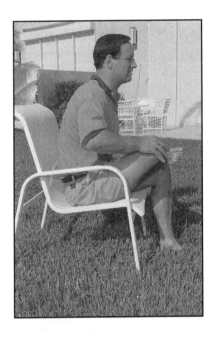

Photo 20-13. Lean your body forward, increasing the intensity of the stretch into your hip and lower back area. This is a Level 2 flexibility position.

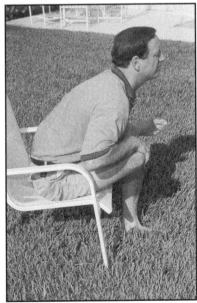

Photo 20-14. As you gain flexibility, you'll be able to lean farther forward. This will maintain your newly improved range of motion in your hips. This is a Level 3 flexibility position.

261

Standing Inner Thigh Stretch

A healthy stretch of your inner thigh muscle helps balance the various muscle groups so they can all work efficiently together. Alternate sides and slowly stretch each leg twice, holding for 15 seconds.

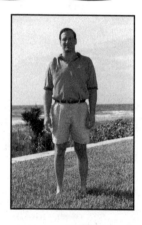

Photo 20-15. Stand up straight and take a few deep breaths.

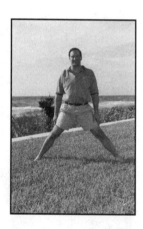

Photo 20-16. Spread your legs wide apart.

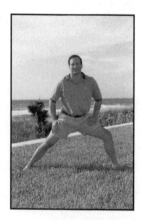

Photo 20-17. Put your hands on your thighs and lean to one side. Point the foot, on the side you want to lean to, toward that direction.

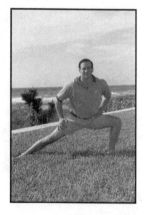

Photo 20-18. Lean all the way to the bent side. Be sure your knee does not go farther than a 90-degree angle.

Frog Stretch

This healthy stretch is for your hip joints and inner thighs. In the advanced position, you'll really create body awareness of your hip joints rotating as the pelvis goes forward. Stretch twice, holding for 15 seconds.

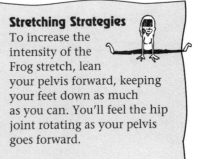
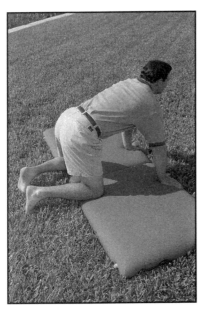

Photo 20-19. Start off on all fours, keeping your back straight.

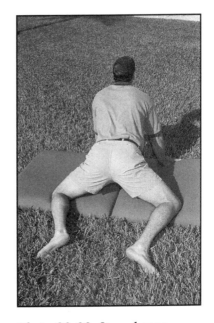

Photo 20-20. Spread your knees as far apart as you can. Your ankles should be inside your knees so you have "frog's legs." Be sure the inside of each ankle touches the ground. To increase the stretch, lean your pelvis forward.

One-Legged Frog Stretch

This healthy stretch will be felt all the way from the inside of the knee up to the inner thigh of the stretched leg. If you're especially tight, you may even feel it in the opposite inner thigh. Alternate and slowly stretch each leg twice, holding for 15 seconds.

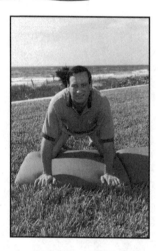

Photo 20-21. Start on your hands and knees.

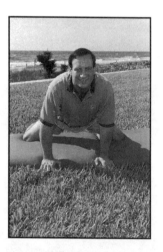

Photo 20-22. Spread your knees as far apart as you can outside your hips.

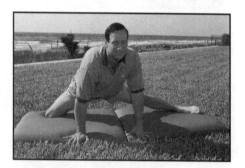

Photo 20-23. Stretch one leg straight out to the side.

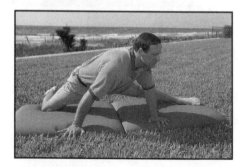

Photo 20-24. Lean your shoulders toward the outstretched leg. Be sure your weight is forward.

Level 1 Triangle Quad Stretch

The quad muscles, the big muscles in front of your thighs, need a good, healthy stretch. You'll feel this from the front of your knee to the front of your hip. Stretch slowly and increase your range of flexibility gradually. Alternate and stretch each leg twice, holding for 15 seconds.

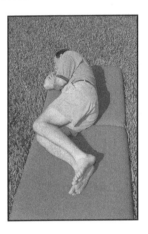

Photo 20-25. Lie on your side with your knees bent.

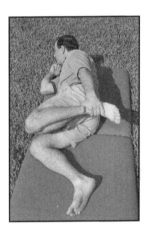

Photo 20-26. Reach back and grab your ankle. Pull it toward your derrière as you keep your knee bent.

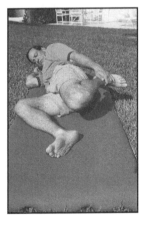

Photo 20-27. Stretch your knee back by pulling it with your hand. Notice that my hip, shoulder, and knee are in a straight line.

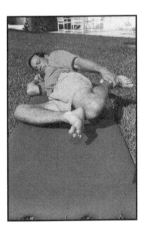

Photo 20-28. Place the heel of the opposite foot on your knee and push the knee back behind the hip. Notice it's still in line with my shoulder.

Advanced Triangle Quad Stretch

This advanced flexibility stretch is done with a towel. I'm using my stretching table but you can use the edge of your bed just as effectively. Alternate and stretch each leg twice, holding for 15 seconds.

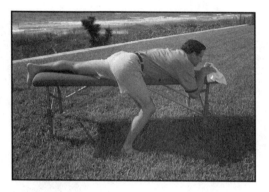

Photo 20-29. Lie down on the bed so that one leg is stretched out on the bed with the other foot on the ground.

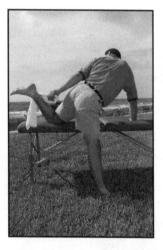

Photo 20-30. Reach back to place the towel around your ankle.

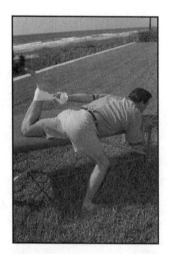

Photo 20-31. Using the towel as a stretching aid, I pull my leg to my derrière.

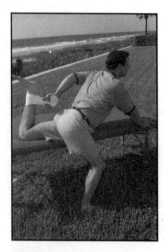

Photo 20-32. Raise your shoulders up to increase the stretch as you pull your leg back with the towel.

Chair Lunge

This three-level stretch helps the front of your quads and the hip. Start with Level 1 and progress as far through the levels as your flexibility will allow. Alternate legs and slowly stretch two times, holding for 15 seconds.

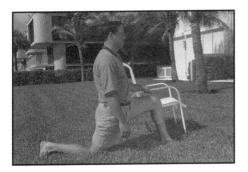

Photo 20-33. Level 1: Bend down on one knee with your leg stretched behind. Your "up leg" should form a 90-degree angle. Push your hips forward.

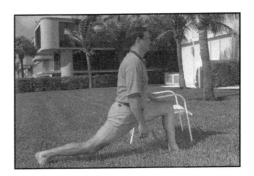

Photo 20-34. Level 2: Raise your back leg up so it's only slightly bent. Push your hips forward.

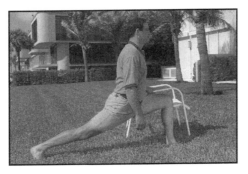

Photo 20-35. Level 3: Straighten your leg as you're pushing your hips and shoulders forward. Keep your shoulders above your hips.

Hamstring Stretch

Hamstrings are the large muscles in the back of your thighs. Depending on your flexibility, choose a level that's comfortable for you. The flexibility self-test may have demonstrated that the muscle is exceptionally tight. If that's the case, begin and stay with Level 1 for a while. Increase your range of motion slowly but steadily. You'll notice any improved flexibility immediately.

Level 1 Hamstring Stretch

Level 1 will provide a good healthy stretch for your hamstrings. It may be all you ever want or need to do. Slowly stretch each leg twice as you alternate them. Hold for 15 seconds.

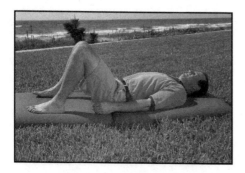

Photo 20-36. Lie on your back with your knees bent.

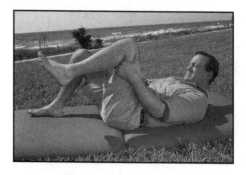

Photo 20-37. Put both hands under the knee of one leg and slowly pull it up toward your hip so the knee forms a 90-degree angle.

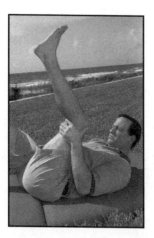

Photo 20-38. Pull your knee toward your chest and slightly straighten your leg. You'll feel the stretch in the center of the hamstring muscle.

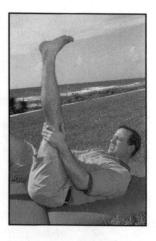

Photo 20-39. Straighten your leg all the way. The stretch will be felt in the hamstring muscle and also behind your knee.

Level 2 Hamstring Stretch

Use a towel to help increase the intensity of the stretch. Begin the same way as Level 1, but wrap a towel around your ankle to provide stretching leverage.

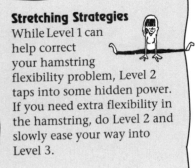

Stretching Strategies
While Level 1 can help correct your hamstring flexibility problem, Level 2 taps into some hidden power. If you need extra flexibility in the hamstring, do Level 2 and slowly ease your way into Level 3.

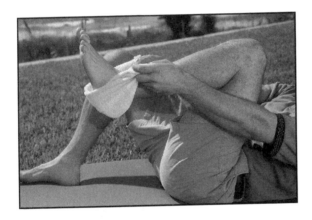

Photo 20-40. Wrap a towel around your heel.

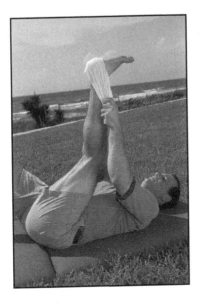

Photo 20-41. Follow all steps of the Level 1 stretch, but use the towel to increase the stretch at the top. Stretch slowly.

Level 3 Hamstring Stretch

I'm using my outside wall for this stretch but most people can use a doorway inside. You want to be able to start with both legs raised, but be able to lower one to the ground. Do this stretch only if you are completely flexible in your hamstrings. Alternate legs and slowly stretch twice, holding for 15 seconds.

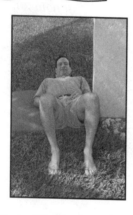

Photo 20-42. I'm lying perpendicular to the wall.

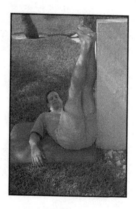

Photo 20-43. As I raise my legs, I'm able to get my derrière very close to the wall.

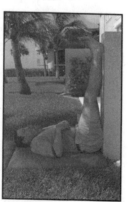

Photo 20-44. I swivel slightly so my legs can go straight up the wall together.

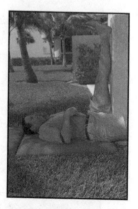

Photo 20-45. I've slowly lowered one leg to the ground while keeping the other up against the wall. You can use a doorway for this.

Butterfly Stretch

The inner thigh receives an outstanding healthy stretch with the Butterfly. Stretch slowly, and don't force yourself into the hold position. Stretch twice, holding for 15 seconds.

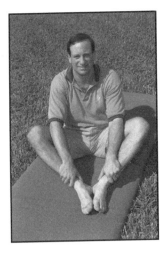

Photo 20-46. Sit with your knees spread apart, heels together. Hold your ankles with your hands.

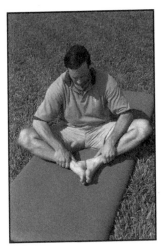

Photo 20-47. Slowly push down on your knees with your elbows.

The Least You Need to Know

➤ It's important to stretch muscle groups to make sure the real cause of the flexibility problem has been discovered and corrected.

➤ Once a muscle is stretched to its proper length, maintaining the muscle's flexibility is your goal.

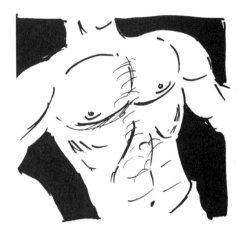

Chapter 21

Healthy Stretching Your Back and Abdomen

In This Chapter

➤ Healthy stretches to improve flexibility in shortened muscles in your back and abdomen

➤ Closely following the photos and instructions will help you obtain maximum results

Back problems rank high on the list of complaints people have. While some cases are the result of damage to the discs or vertebrae, many complaints are actually muscle-related. Healthy stretching the muscles of the back and abdomen helps prevent the tight muscles from pressing on nerves, causing muscle groups to tighten as a protection against further injury.

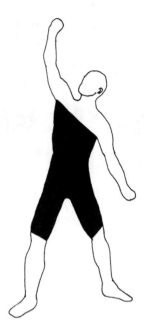

Figure 21-1. Abdomen muscle groups.

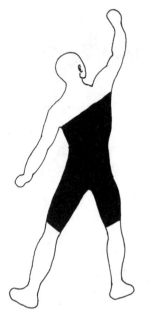

Figure 21-2. Back muscle groups.

Chris's Concerns
If you are currently undergoing medical treatment for a back problem, do not do any of these stretches without discussing them with your doctor first. If you have been injured and did not consult a doctor, please do so before beginning any healthy stretching.

If the Chapter 1 flexibility self-test discovered that your back and abdomen need flexibility improvement, try the healthy stretches in this chapter as well as those in Chapter 20.

One Knee to Chest

This lower back stretch is an easy way to begin. You'll feel the stretch in the back of your hamstrings and your lower back. Alternate legs and slowly stretch twice, holding for 15 seconds.

Stretching Strategies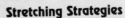

If you feel a tightness or pinching in the front of your leg, you also need to healthy stretch other areas. Chapter 20 refers you to stretches for the quad muscles and hips. Very often the problem is not where you think it is. In this case, your tightness is most likely being caused by inflexibility in the quads and hip.

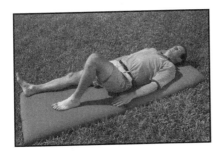

Photo 21-1. Lie on your back with one knee bent.

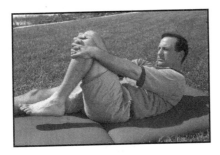

Photo 21-2. Reach up and hold your knee with both hands.

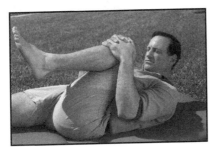

Photo 21-3. Stretch your knee toward your chest.

Two Knees to Chest

This is a massage stretch. Rocking back and forth warms up the spinal erector muscles that go up the spine. Stretch slowly to the roll position and rock back and forth, five times.

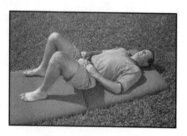

Photo 21-4. Lie on your back with both knees bent.

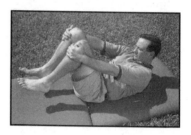

Photo 21-5. Reach up and hold your knees with both hands.

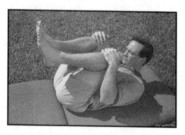

Photo 21-6. Stretch your knees up toward your chest.

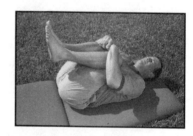

Photo 21-7. Stretch your knees to your chest with your head flat.

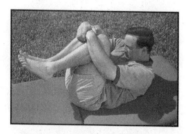

Photo 21-8. Rocking your head up toward your knees creates a rolling massage for your back muscles.

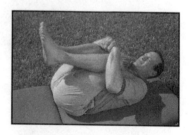

Photo 21-9. Rock back with your hands still holding your knees to your chest.

Sitting Lower Back Stretch

This is a Level 3 healthy stretch. Only stretch to the level your flexibility permits. Hold that position for 15 seconds and do the stretch twice. As your flexibility increases over time, stretch your way to the next level. The stretch is felt in your lower back. To really benefit from the Sitting Lower Back stretch, stretch slowly into the Level 1 position. If you already feel tightness, that's the level to stay at for a while. Once the tightness is stretched out, over time, proceed to the next level. *Never bounce your way into the position.* Slowly stretch, feeling the muscles lengthen during the 15-second hold.

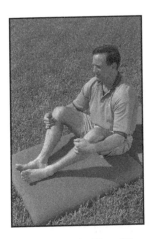

Photo 21-10. Sit with your knees spread apart and hold onto your knees.

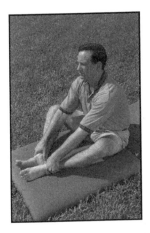

Photo 21-11. Level 1: Stretch down slowly and hold your ankles. Keep your back straight.

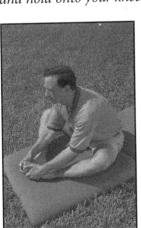

Photo 21-12. Level 2: Stretch slowly as you put your hands on your feet. Keep your back straight as you bend forward.

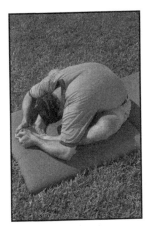

Photo 21-13. Level 3: Advanced flexibility. Slowly stretch all the way forward.

Chris's Concerns

If you are experiencing shoulder problems or know that you have a shoulder injury, do not do this stretch. It requires putting some weight on your shoulders for leverage.

Shoulder Back Roll

This Level 3 stretch will help increase the flexibility of your mid- and lower back. In Level 3, the oblique muscles on the side of your abdomen will also feel the stretch. Only stretch as far as is comfortable. As your flexibility increases, you can stretch your way to the next level. Do this stretch on a padded floor or on the grass. Slowly stretch each side twice, holding for 15 seconds.

Photo 21-14. Start on your hands and knees.

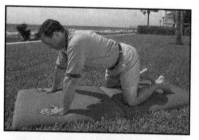

Photo 21-15. Level 1: Ease down and lie on one shoulder, bracing your body with the other arm.

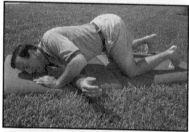

Photo 21-16. Level 2: Put your hand behind your back and stretch back. You should feel your upper torso start to twist and your lower and mid-back stretching.

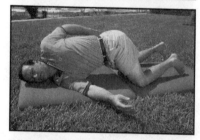

Photo 21-17. Level 3: Stretch your free arm back behind you. This increases the stretch so you feel it in your back and your oblique muscles.

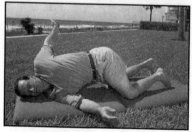

Torso Stretch

This is an excellent healthy stretch for your upper back. If you're especially tight, you'll also feel the stretch in your lower back. Change positions and stretch each side twice, holding for 15 seconds. You do not have to use a palm tree for this healthy stretch—use any fixed object you can hold onto, like a doorknob, tree, or car bumper. Stretch each side twice, holding for 15 seconds.

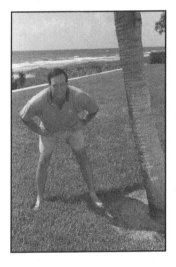 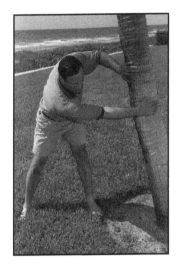 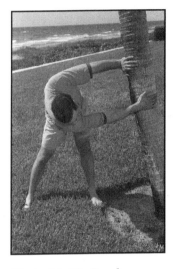

Photo 21-18. Stand sideways to whatever you choose to use for stretching help. Bend over, hands on thighs.

Photo 21-19. Reach over and grab, in my case, the tree, with your lower hand. Brace yourself with your other hand.

Photo 21-20. Bend over so your shoulders are the same height as your waist. Straighten your top arm by pushing with the top arm and pulling with the lower arm.

Level 1 Two Knees Over

This is the Level 1 stretch for your back and abdomen. If you can comfortably hold the stretch with your shoulders flat on the ground, proceed to the next level. Hold for 15 seconds for each side. Stretch each side twice.

Photo 21-21. Lie on your back with your knees bent.

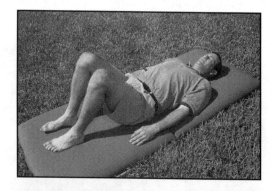

Photo 21-22. With your knees together, slowly roll to one side. Keep your shoulders flat.

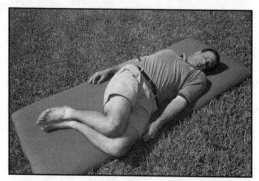

Photo 21-23. Stretch to the other side.

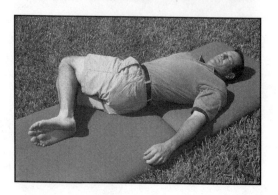

Levels 2 and 3 One Knee Over

Here is the more intensive healthy stretch for the lower back and abdomen. Once you can easily hold the position in Level 2, continue on as you stretch to Level 3. Level 3 will also stretch your hamstrings. Slowly stretch each side twice, holding for 15 seconds.

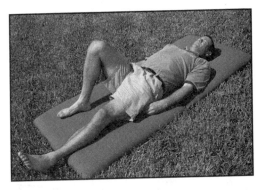

Photo 21-24. Lie on your back with one knee bent.

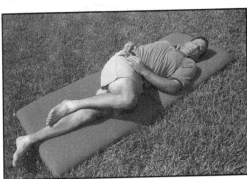

Photo 21-25. Keeping your shoulders flat, stretch the bent knee over the straight one.

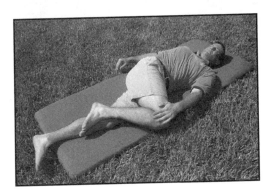

Photo 21-26. Level 2: Reach down and put your hand on the crossed-over knee. Push down on the knee, still keeping your shoulders flat.

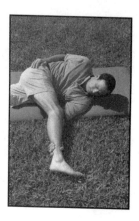

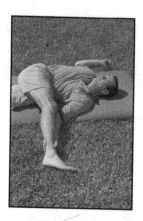

Photo 21-27. Level 3: From the crossed-over position, stretch your leg as it's straightened to form a 90-degree angle with the other leg. Reach your hand down to hold your ankle.

Photo 21-28. Lay your shoulders back down to increase the stretch. You'll feel this from your hamstrings to the sides of your back. Keep your knees slightly bent.

Side Overhead Arch

This healthy stretch is a nice final one to do for the muscles of your back, abdomen, and arms. Slowly stretch yourself over and form an arch. You'll feel the stretch in the sides and front of your abdomen. Reverse positions as you stretch each side twice.

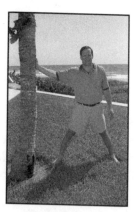

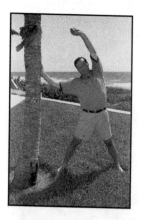

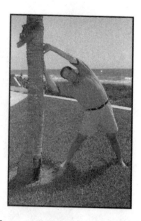

Photo 21-29. Stand an arm's length to the side of something you can hold onto. I'm using my palm tree but you can use a door or pole. Spread your legs more than shoulder-width apart.

Photo 21-30. Feel the stretch as you reach over your head toward your supporting hand.

Photo 21-31. Keep stretching as far as you can comfortably go. Touching the tree is your ultimate goal.

The Least You Need to Know

➤ Healthy stretching helps prevent tight muscles from pressing on nerves, causing other muscle groups to tighten.

➤ Healthy stretching your back and abdomen provides energy while protecting against potential injury.

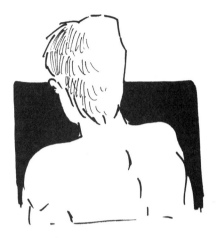

Chapter 22

Healthy Stretching Your Shoulders and Neck

In This Chapter

➤ Healthy stretches for flexibility problems in your shoulders and neck

➤ Healthy stretch away tight muscles caused by tension in your daily life

The tension of daily life seems to show itself in our shoulders and neck, as illustrated in Figure 22-1. Very often neck flexibility problems are caused by tightness that starts in our shoulders. These healthy stretches are designed to educate the muscles to return to their proper lengths, releasing the tightness.

*Figure 22-1.
Shoulders and neck
muscle groups.*

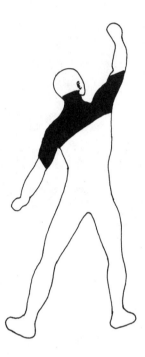

As muscles lengthen, the tightness and tension are stretched away. If you've been tight for a while, you'll almost immediately notice the difference. The area will become warm and you'll start feeling relaxation creeping in. Stay as relaxed as possible when doing these stretches. Take deep breaths to help ease the tension away.

Stretching Strategies
The neck stretches are in three Levels. If you're getting relief from Level 1, then stay with it. If you desire additional stretching for your neck, do Level 2. Level 3 is done on the ground so you may want to do this one at home at night.

Level 1 Neck Side-to-Side Stretch

We'll begin with a nice relaxing stretch for the neck. Take some deep breaths, smile, and stretch slowly from side to side. Try and keep your shoulders level as you stretch from side to side. Do this stretch three times for each side, holding for 15 seconds.

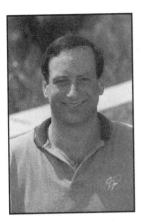

Photo 22-1. Begin by looking straight ahead.

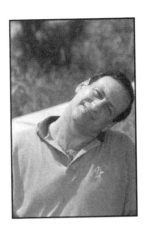

Photo 22-2. Slowly stretch your head toward one shoulder.

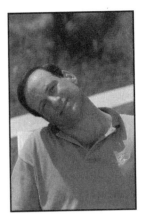

Photo 22-3. Stretch to the other side. If you want to increase the stretch, slowly lower your shoulder down on the opposite side.

Level 2 Seated Neck Stretch

This is a more intensive healthy stretch for your neck. It's great to do if you're getting stiff while at work, in your car, or on a plane. It can be done almost anywhere you can sit. The stretch is felt in your neck and into the side of your arm. Alternate sides for the stretch. Do it twice for each side, holding for 15 seconds.

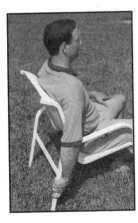

Photo 22-4. Sit in a chair and reach down and grab the lowest part of the chair you can reach.

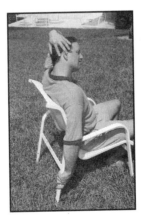

Photo 22-5. Reach your free hand over and place it on the opposite side of your head.

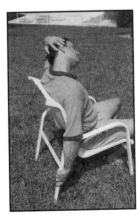

Photo 22-6. Use your hand on your head to stretch your neck slowly away from the hand that's holding the chair.

287

Level 3 Back Neck Stretch

This healthy stretch, done on your back, really increases the ability for you to stretch all the built-up tension away. You may want to save it for later in the day. Stretch each side twice, holding for 15 seconds.

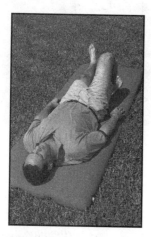

Photo 22-7. Lie on your back and bend one knee.

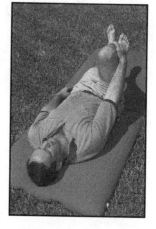

Photo 22-8. Hold onto the knee with your hand from the same side.

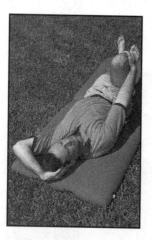

Photo 22-9. Place your free hand on the opposite side of your head.

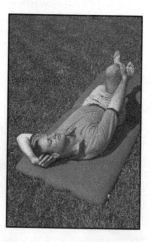

Photo 22-10. Stretch your head away from the hand holding your knee. Pushing your knee away will increase the stretch even more.

Chin-Ups Stretch

This healthy stretch is wonderful for both the front and back of your neck. Start with Level 2 and then progress to Level 3 as your flexibility increases. Do the stretch twice and hold for 15 seconds.

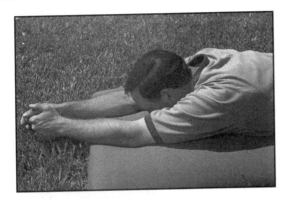

Photo 22-11. Lie face down with your head straight. Stretch your arms in front of you.

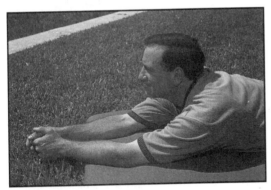

Photo 22-12. Level 2: Stretch your chin up as far as you can.

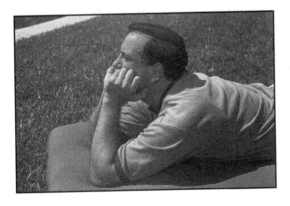

Photo 22-13. Level 3: Bend your elbows and place your hands under your chin. Push your chin up and out, increasing the stretch.

Shoulder Arm Across the Body Stretch

This healthy stretch was part of the Chapter 1 flexibility self-test. How far were you able to stretch your arm across your chest? Now you can increase shoulder flexibility. Stretch twice for each side, holding for 15 seconds.

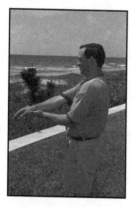

Photo 22-14. Stand straight and bring your arm across your body, parallel to the ground. Hold it with your opposite hand.

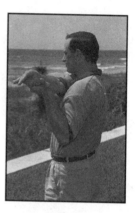

Photo 22-15. Pull the hand toward your body as far as you can go. Hold for 15 seconds.

Biceps Stretch

This healthy stretch works on the front of your shoulder down into your elbow. Stretch slowly twice, holding for 15 seconds.

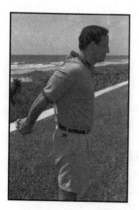

Photo 22-16. Stand straight and grasp your hands behind your back.

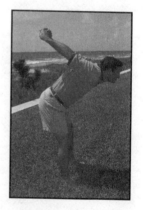

Photo 22-17. Slightly bend over and bring your arms up.

Triceps Stretch

If you do the biceps stretch for the front of your shoulder, also do the triceps stretch for the back of your shoulder to balance the shoulder. It's a two-level stretch starting with Level 2. Level 3 provides additional stretching by leaning. Alternate and slowly stretch each side twice, holding for 15 seconds.

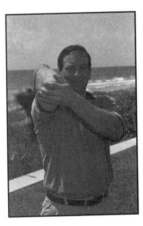

Photo 22-18. Bend one arm straight back. Put your opposite hand on your elbow.

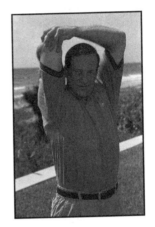

Photo 22-19. Level 2: Stretch your elbow back by pulling it with your hand. You'll feel the stretch in your arm up to your elbow. Hold for 15 seconds.

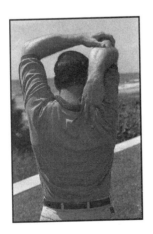

Photo 22-20. This is how it looks from behind.

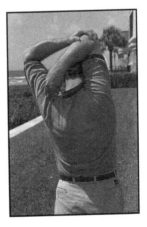

Photo 22-21. Level 3: To increase the stretch so that you feel it in the triceps muscle that connects to the shoulder and elbow, pull your elbow slightly across your back.

291

Sleeper Stretch

This is my favorite healthy stretch. You should feel this in your rotator cuff, the muscle that goes up over your shoulder from front to back. Stretch each shoulder twice, holding for 15 seconds.

If you feel the stretch only in the front of your shoulder, stop. The elbow needs to be repositioned up or down so you can feel the stretch in your back. It's important to keep your shoulder down; that's why your chin is pressing on it.

Photo 22-22. Lie down on your side and put your chin on your shoulder.

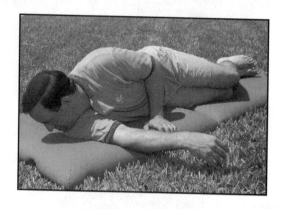

Photo 22-23. This is a close-up view of how your chin should be on your shoulder.

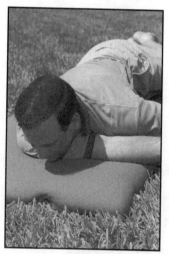

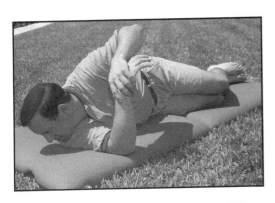

Photo 22-24. Bend your arm that will be stretched and put your opposite hand on the back of the wrist.

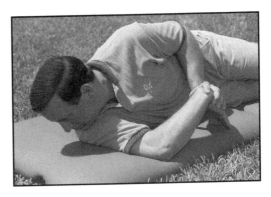

Photo 22-25. Your arm stretches down as the hand pushes it. As your goal, try to touch the floor or ground with your fingers.

The Least You Need to Know

➤ Very often, neck flexibility problems begin as a result of tightness in the shoulders.

➤ Try to relax while doing the neck and shoulder healthy stretches. Take deep breaths to help ease away tension.

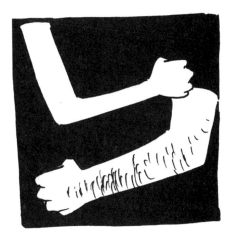

Chapter 23

Healthy Stretching Your Elbows and Wrists

In This Chapter

➤ Healthy stretches for flexibility problems in your elbows and wrists

➤ Healthy stretching helps prevent carpal tunnel syndrome

Most people never think about stretching their elbows and wrists. Or if they do, it's only to crack their knuckles. But think about how often you use them—almost all the time. Healthy stretching will keep your elbows and wrists flexible and even help prevent some problems like carpal tunnel syndrome.

These healthy stretches will only take a few minutes to do. The muscle groups go all the way up to the deltoid muscles in your shoulder. The biceps and triceps muscles of the upper arm actually connect below the elbow. The muscles of the lower arm connect below the wrist and above the elbow, as in Figure 23-1.

Figure 23-1. The muscle groups of the wrists and elbows.

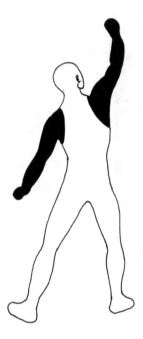

Straight Elbow Stretch

Most of us keep our elbows slightly bent all the time. A good healthy stretch is one that stretches your elbow out straight. You'll feel the stretch in the front of your elbow. Stretch each elbow twice, holding for 15 seconds.

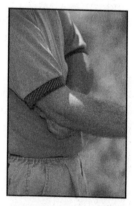

Photo 23-1. Put your opposite fist under your elbow. Your arm should be slightly bent.

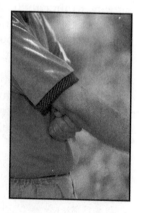

Photo 23-2. Straighten your arm out and push up with your fist.

Table Elbow Stretch

Use a desk, table, or the ground for this elbow stretch. Alternate elbows and stretch twice, holding for 15 seconds.

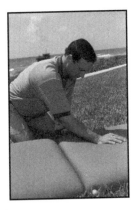

Photo 23-3. Put your hand down with your elbow slightly bent. Put your opposite fist under the elbow.

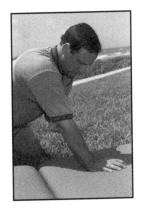

Photo 23-4. Straighten your arm as you push against your elbow.

Pointed Elbow Stretch

This healthy stretch works on several connecting muscle groups. Since you just stretched your elbow back, you need to stretch in the other direction to balance the muscle groups, helping the elbow flexibly rotate. Stretch each elbow twice and hold for 15 seconds.

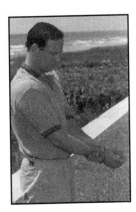

Photo 23-5. Hold your wrist with the opposite hand.

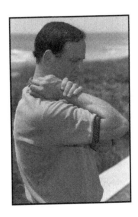

Photo 23-6. Stretch your elbow up to shoulder height as you bend your elbow.

Wrist Twist Stretch Down

You can do these twist stretches with your elbow bent or straight. I'm demonstrating it with a bent elbow. Alternate wrists and twist slowly twice, holding for 15 seconds.

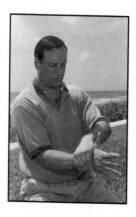

Photo 23-7. Raise one arm parallel to the ground at your waist. The thumb should be straight up. Hold the wrist with your other hand.

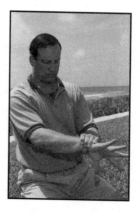

Photo 23-8. Using your holding hand, twist the wrist so the thumb goes down. You'll feel the stretch in the top and outside parts of your elbow.

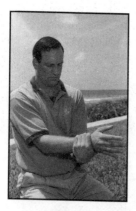

Photo 23-9. Now put the opposite hand under the wrist.

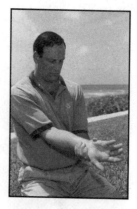

Photo 23-10. Twist slowly in the opposite direction, with your palm going away from you. The stretch can be felt on the inside and front of your elbow.

Wrist and Elbow Stretch

This healthy Level 1 stretch works on your wrists and elbows. It's also good prevention against "tennis elbow." Do it slowly and feel the muscles stretching. Stretch each arm twice, holding for 15 seconds.

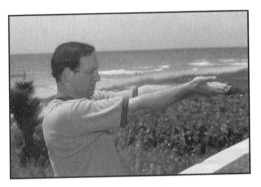

Photo 23-11. Pick up your arms and hold them straight out in front. Palms should be facing up. Take one hand and place it palm to palm on the other hand.

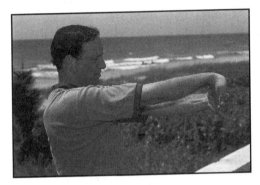

Photo 23-12. Push the top palm down stretching the wrist back, keeping the elbow straight. You'll feel the stretch in the wrist through the forearm.

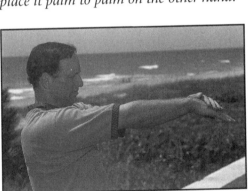

Photo 23-13. Now turn one palm facing down and place the other palm on the back of the opposite hand.

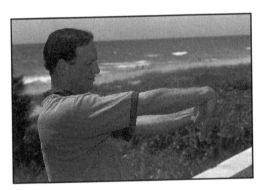

Photo 23-14. Stretch the palm down, pushing it with the top hand. You'll feel the stretch in the top of your wrist and outside of your elbow.

Pushing Wrist Stretches

This series of healthy stretches uses part of the weight of your body to stretch the wrists. You start by getting on your hands and knees. Stretch each direction twice, holding for 15 seconds. The Pushing Wrist stretches are a Level 2 stretch. If you want to intensify the stretch to Level 3, just lean slowly back. Healthy stretching allows you to control the amount of stretch you want.

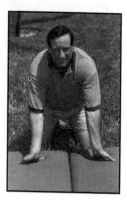

Photo 23-15. Turn your hands so your palms are down but your fingers point toward you. Place them on a padded surface or on the floor in front of you.

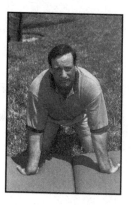

Photo 23-16. Press your wrists into the pad or floor. You'll feel the stretch through your wrists into the front of your elbow.

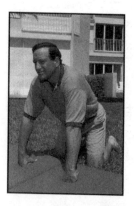

Photo 23-17. Put the back of your hands down with your palms up, fingers pointed toward you.

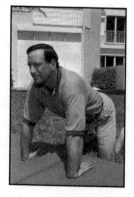

Photo 23-18. Push your wrists down into the pad or floor, while keeping your elbows straight. You'll feel the stretch in the front of your wrists.

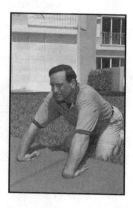

Photo 23-19. The Level 3 stretch occurs as you slowly lean back control-ling the amount of stretch.

Side Wrist Stretches

This healthy stretch works on the wrists with a side-to-side motion. Slowly stretch from one side to the other twice, holding for 15 seconds.

Stretching Strategies
This series of side-to-side wrist stretches will eliminate any remaining tightness you may still have in your wrists. If you don't feel anything, you've been really working on improving your flexibility.

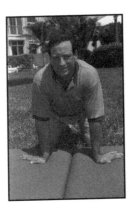

Photo 23-20. Start on your hands and knees. Place your wrists, palms down, fingers pointing out to the sides.

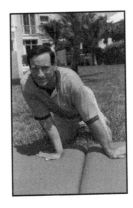

Photo 23-21. Stretch to one side slowly. You'll feel if you have any tightness.

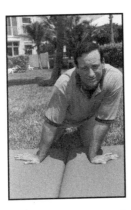

Photo 23-22. Stretch slowly to the other side.

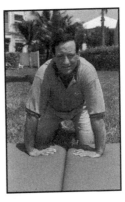

Photo 23-23. Now turn your fingers so they point toward each other.

301

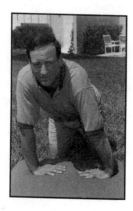

Photo 23-24. Stretch slowly to one side and you should feel some stretching in your elbows and wrists, maybe even slightly in the shoulder.

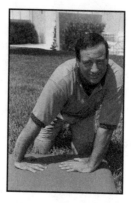

Photo 23-25. Slowly stretch to the other side. You should feel some stretching in your wrists, elbows, and maybe even your shoulder.

The Least You Need to Know

➤ Some of the muscle groups of the elbows are connected to the shoulders.

➤ Other muscle groups of the elbows are connected to the wrists.

Glossary

15-second hold   Healthy stretching a muscle for 15 seconds; helps re-educate muscles back to their proper lengths.

Achilles tendon   The large tendon that connects the calf muscle to the heel.

Ball and socket joint   A joint in which one bone is ball-shaped to rotate in the socket of the other bone.

Body awareness   A developed sense and feel for what the body is doing.

Body compensation   Adjustments the body makes for loss of flexibility.

Bursitis   A painful condition of moveable joints.

C-shape   An incorrect rounded shape of the spine.

Carpal tunnel syndrome   A painful condition of the hand and wrist brought on by repetitive movements.

Cartilage   Found in moveable joints for cushioning and protection.

Contracting   For the purposes of this Guide, it means a voluntary tightening of a muscle.

Derrière   Butt; behind; bottom. Gluteus maximus muscles.

Fatigued muscles   When a muscle fatigues, it actually shortens.

Femur   The large bone in the upper leg.

Flexibility   The ability of your body to move freely.

Hamstrings   The large muscle in the back of your upper leg.

Hinge joint   Allows the bones to move in one plane only. Elbows and knees are examples.

Hip rotator muscles   A small group of muscles that move the foot in and out.

Joint   The point where bones are connected to each other.

Ligaments   Tough bands of tissue that connect bones together.

Limited flexibility   Restricted rotational movement.

Muscle spasm   The immediate shortening of the muscle to protect itself.

Muscle strain   A slight tearing of the muscle.

Overuse syndrome   An injury created by performing repetitive activity for a long period of time.

Pigeon-toed   Toes point inward, usually as a result of inner thigh tightness.

Quadriceps   The large muscles in the front of your upper leg.

Range of motion   A way of measuring the flexibility of a joint.

Rotational flexibility   Body movement in circles within our joints.

S-shape   The correct curvature of the spine.

Scar tissue   New tissue that knits a torn muscle.

Shin splints   A painful condition of the lower leg that can be helped by stretching.

Spinal disc   Cartilage located between the vertebrae to cushion them during movement.

Spine   Twenty-four separate bones called vertebrae.

Stretching balance   Muscles on both sides of the body are of equal length.

Tendons   Tissue that connects muscles to bones.

Tennis elbow   Inflammation of the tendons on the outside of the lower arm.

VCIF   Vicious cycle of inflexibility—fatiguing of an already shortened muscle.

Index

Symbols

15-second hold, 303
    stretching, 47-48

A

abdominal stretches
    Seated Back stretch, 99
    Sitting Twist stretch, 100
Accelerator stretch (driving),
    151
Achilles tendon, 303
    stretching, 180
address position (golf), 162
Advanced Triangle Quad
    stretch (quadriceps), 266
aerobic sports and leisure
    activities, 27
airplane stretches
    Banking Rotation stretch,
        142
    comfort guidelines, 140
    Fighter Pilot stretch, 141
    Flaps-Up Arm stretch, 141
    Landing Gear Neck stretch,
        142
    Landing Gear Up stretch,
        146
    Serving-Tray, Shoulder-Blade
        stretch, 144
    Tail-Section stretch, 144
animals, stretching instincts,
    58, 178

ankles
    flexibility, testing, 13
    ligament damage, 30
    muscle support, 30
    stretches
        Ankle Rotation stretch,
            253
        Ankle stretcher, 172
        tennis, 251
        troubleshooting, 49
arm stretches
    Backward Arm Conditioner
        stretch, 131-132
    Biceps Fence stretch, 171-172
    Cross-Body stretch, 236-237
    Double-Handed stretch, 130
    First Serve stretch, 170
    Flaps-Up Arm stretch, 141
    Hands Up stretch, 78
    Head Rest Arm stretch, 149
    One Arm Seat stretch, 150
    Standing Shoulder stretch,
        235
    Steering-Wheel Twist
        stretch, 147
arthritis, causes, 124
athletes
    and record-breaking perfor-
        mances, 199
    as role models to children,
        221
    body awareness, 198
    effects of stretching, 43-45
    injuries and vicious cycle of
        inflexibility (VCIF), 180
    legs, stretching misconcep-
        tions, 178
automobiles, see driving
    stretches

B

back
    anatomy
        discs, 140
        spine, 140
        vertebrae, 140
    damage
        discs, 273-274
        vertebrae, 273-274
    flexibility, troubleshoot-
        ing, 49
    gardener stretches
        Back Planter stretch, 132
        Both Sides Body Condi-
            tioner stretch, 134
        Hamstring Planter
            stretch, 134
    injury prevention, 273-274
    stretches
        Back Arch stretch, 58-59
        Back Bend Over stretch,
            210
        Back Racket stretch, 167
        Back Rockers stretch, 95
        Bend Over Twist
            stretch, 66
        Extended Side-to-Side
            stretch, 94
        for gardeners stretch, 132
        Front Bend stretch, 64
        Gentle Back stretch, 105
        Lumbar Roll stretch, 150
        One Knee Over stretch,
            281
        One Knee to Chest
            stretch, 275

Shoulder Back Roll stretch, 278
Side Overhead Arch stretch, 282
Side Quad stretch, 214
Sitting Lower-Back stretch, 277
Squat and Sit stretch, 80
Tail-Section stretch, 144
Togetherness Side-to-Side stretch, 97
Torso Press-Up stretch, 60
Torso stretch, 279
Two Knees Over stretch, 280
Two Knees to Chest stretch, 276
work-site stretches
Pipe Bender stretch, 136
Pipe Twister stretch, 138
stretching precautions, doctor consultation, 273-274
Back Bend-Over stretch (pregnancy), 210
Back Leaner stretch (children), 226
Back Neck stretch, 288
Back Planter stretch (gardeners), 132
Back Racket stretch (tennis), 167
Back Rocker stretch (nighttime), 95
backaches, treating, 30
Backhand Push stretch (carpal tunnel syndrome), 114
Backward Arm Conditioner stretch (physical labor), 131-132
ball and socket joints, 303
moveable joint types, 38-40
Banking Rotation stretch (airplanes), 142
Bend Over Twist stretch, 66
Biceps Fence stretch (tennis), 171-172
Biceps stretch (shoulders), 290
biceps tendonitis, 131
Birdie Hip stretch (golf), 158
Black Diamond stretch (skiing), 205

blood
pooling in lower extremities, 116
pressure, waking up, 59
warmth and flexibility, 64
body
asymmetry, 9-10
awareness, 198, 303
compensation, 303
energy through stretches, 74
getting out of bed, 57
muscles, work process, 37
overcompensating, 6
postures
examining, 6-11
"Leaning Tower of Pisa," 9-10
side view, 10-11
"Statue of Liberty," 6
record-breaking performances, 199
symmetry, 6
types
Football Players, 25
Marathon Runners, 25
range of flexibility, 24-25
Supermodels, 26
Workout Woman, 25-26
bones
connective tissues, 34-35
femur, 34-35
fractures, rehabilitating, 23
functions, 34-35
ilium, 34-35
joints, 23, 38-40
ligament strains, 24
number in human body, 34-35
pelvis, 34-35
relationships to muscles, 34
tendons, 24
tibia, 34-35
Both Sides Body Conditioner stretch (gardeners), 134
bouncing during stretches, 182
bridge of energy, 74
bursitis, 303
joints, 38-40
Butterfly stretch (hamstrings), 271

C

C-shape (spinal column), 303
Calves Pole stretch (runners), 180
calf stretches
Standing Calf stretch, 246-247
Standing Heel and Calf stretch, 248
Campfire Sitting stretch (children), 228
Cannon Ball stretch (children), 225
carpal tunnel syndrome, 113, 303
as source of workers' compensation claims, 113-114
ergonomic keyboard replacement, 114
preventative measures, 114
rest periods, 114
stretches
Backhand Push, 114
Wrist Relievers, 115-116
World Health Organization (WHO), 113-114
cars, *see* driving stretches
Cart Quad stretch (golf), 157
cartilage, 303
joints, 38-40
Cat and Dog stretch, 58-59
Chair lunge stretch (quadriceps), 267-271
children
athletes as role models, 221
flexibility
benefits, 221
problems
hip flexor problems, 219-220
Osgood-Slaghter disease, 220
puberty, 220
sedentary lifestyles
inflexible muscles, 220-221
lethargy, 220-221
self-esteem problems, 220-221

stretches
    Back Leaner stretch, 226
    Campfire Sitting stretch, 228
    Cannon Ball stretch, 225
    Hamstring stretch, 227
    Hands Above the Head stretch, 222
    Neck stretch, 230
    One-Foot stretch, 222
    Side stretch, 224
    Soccer stretch, 223
    Swordsmen lunge, 229-230
stretching
    encouraging daily regimen, 220
    parental communication, 227
chin exercises for facial muscles, 63
Chin-Ups stretch (neck), 289
clubhead speed in golf swing, 156-157
cold temperatures, proper warm-up of muscles, 199
comfort guidelines, airplane stretches, 140
compensating for vacationing muscles, 40-41
"compilation of compensations" (golf swings), 156
computers and carpal tunnel syndrome, 113-114
couch potato lifestyle, 29
cracking necks, 18
cross country skiing, *see* skiing
Crossover stretch (pregnancy), 212
Cross-Body Arm stretch (senior citizens), 236-237
Curtain Call stretch (nighttime), 107
cyclist injuries
    hip joints, 179
    quadricep tightness, 179

D

Diamond stretch (nighttime), 104-105
discs, 140

doctor consultation, 45
    back stretching, 273-274
    senior citizen stretching programs, 233
Door stretch (driving), 148
driving stretches, 147
    Accelerator stretch, 151
    Door stretch, 148
    Head-Rest Arm stretch, 149
    Lumbar Roll stretch, 150
    One-Arm Seat stretch, 150
    Steering-Wheel Twist stretch, 147
Dynamic Quad stretch (runners), 183

E

Eagle Inner Thigh stretch (golf), 159
Ear to Shoulder stretch, 88
Edge Sharpener stretch (skiing), 200-201
elbows
    flexibility, testing, 16
    stretches
        Over Grip Net stretch, 169
        Pointed Elbow stretch, 297
        Straight Elbow stretch, 296
        Table Elbow stretch, 297
        Tennis Elbow stretch, 299
        Under Grip Net stretch, 168
        Wrist Twist stretch, 298
En Garde lunges (senior citizens), 237
endurance sports, 26-27
energy stretches
    Frog Squat stretch, 75
    Front Hip Flexor stretch, 77-78
    Front Squat stretch, 74-75
    Hands Up stretch, 78
    rebuilding stretch, 74
    Side Bend stretch, 78
    Squat and Sit stretch, 80
    Squat and Twist stretch, 81
    Squat lunge, 76
    Standing Calf stretch, 77

ergonomic keyboards and carpal tunnel syndrome, 113-114
evaluating flexibility, 19
examining body postures, 6-11
exercising and stretching
    accompanying exercises, 46-47
    guidelines, 47
Extended Back stretcher (nighttime), 92-94
Extended Side-to-Side stretch (nighttime), 94

F

facial muscles
    chin exercises, 63
    toning, 62-63
Faldo, Nick (pro golfer), on importance of stretching, 155-156
fascicles (muscles), 36-37
fatigued muscles, 23, 27
feet
    blood pooling in lower extremities, 116
    shoe purchases, 116
    stretches, 252
        Ankle Rotation stretch, 253
        Edge Sharpener stretch, 200-201
        Toe and Foot stretch, 252
femur bone, 34, 185, 303
Fighter Pilot stretch (airplanes), 141
First Serve stretch (tennis), 170
Flaps-Up Arm stretch (airplanes), 141
flexibility
    adults versus children, 40
    and blood warmth, 64
    and swimming, 193
    and vacationing muscles, 40-41
    body, overcompensating, 6
    body types, 4
        Football Players, 25
        Marathon Runners, 25
        ranges, 24-25
        Workout Woman, 25-26

childhood problems
    Osgood-Slaghter disease, 220
    tight hamstrings, 219-220
during pregnancy, 210
hips, 30
in children, benefits, 221
in pro athletes, 44-45
inactive muscles, building, 41
leisure activities
    aerobic sports, 27
    couch potatoes, 29
    endurance sports, 26-27
    Weekend Warriors, 28
limited (knees), 12
mogul skiing, 203
necks, cracking, 18
past injuries, 23-24
problems, identifying, 45
relationship of muscles to bones, 34
results, evaluating, 19
sitting position (pain), 30
specialists, searching, 31
standing position (pain), 30
Supermodel body type, 26
testing
    ankles, 13
    elbows, 16
    hips, 13-14
    knees, 11-12
    neck, 18
    shoulders, 14-16
    wrists, 17
troubleshooting, 49
flexibility specialists, searching, 31
football players and flexibility, 25
footstep patterns
    "pigeon-toed"
        causes, 5
        in athletes, 5
        straightening, 5
    "waddling duck"
        causes, 5
        hip tightness, 5
        straightening, 5
fractures
    casts, 23
    physician examination, 24
    rehabilitating, 23

Freestyle stretch (swimming), 194
Frog Squat stretch, 75
Frog stretch
    swimming, 196
    thighs, 263
Front Bend stretch, 64
Front Hip Flexor stretch, 77-78
Front Squat stretch, 74-75
Full Pretzel stretch (hips), 258

G

gardener stretches, 132
    Back Planter stretch, 132
    Both Sides Body Conditioner stretch, 134
    Hamstring Planter stretch, 134-136
Gentle Back stretch (nighttime), 105
gliding joints, 38-40
golf
    address position, 162
    Faldo, Nick (pro golfer), on importance of stretching, 155-156
    hip rotation, 162
    importance of proper stretching, 155-156
    mental approach, 162
    muscles
        hip flexors, 156-157
        quadriceps, 156-157
    rotational flexibility, 155-157
    stretches
        Birdie Hip stretch, 158
        Cart Quad stretch, 157
        Eagle Inner Thigh stretch, 159
        Long Driver Shoulder stretch, 160-161
    swings
        as "compilation of compensations," 156
        clubhead speed, 156-157

H

Hamstring Bench stretch (tennis), 174
Hamstring Conditioner stretch (physical labor), 126
hamstring muscles, 54
Hamstring Planter stretch (gardeners), 134-136
Hamstring Standing stretch (office) 120-121
Hamstring stretch
    children, 227
    pregnancy, 216
Hamstring Striding stretch (runners), 182
hamstrings, 267-271, 303
    stretches
        Butterfly stretch, 271
        Level 1 Hamstring stretch, 268
        Level 2 Hamstring stretch, 269
        Level 3 Hamstring stretch, 270
Hands Above the Head stretch (children), 222
Hands Up stretch, 78
Head Forward and Back stretch, 87
Head-Rest Arm stretch (driving), 149
Head Rotation stretch, 89
heart muscles, 36-37
hinge joints, 303
    moveable joint type, 38-40
hip replacement surgery in senior citizens, 240
hip rotator muscles, 303
hips
    femur bone, 185
    flexibility
        in knees, 30
        limited, 13-14
        testing, 13-14
    locked, 232
    replacement surgery in senior citizens, 240
    rotation (golf) 162
    stretches
        Black Diamond stretch, 205
        Full Pretzel stretch, 258

Hamstring Standing stretch, 120-121
Modified Pretzel stretch, 257
Partner Hip stretch, 218
Quad Muscle Wake-Up stretch, 118
Seated Hip stretch, 260
Sitting Hip stretch, 116
Sitting Outside Hip stretch, 117
Standing Hip stretch, 185, 204
Standing Inner-Thigh stretch, 262
Standing Shoulder stretch, 240
Wall Side Bend stretch, 68
tightness, 274
Horizontal Towel stretch, 70

I

identifying flexibility problems, 45
ilium (bones), 34
inactive muscles, stretching, 41
injuries
    animals, stretching preventatives, 178
    ankles, 179
    flexibility, effects on, 23-24
    fractures, 23-24
    hip
        flexors, 179
        joints, 179
    knees, 179
    ligament strains, 23-24
    muscles in cold temperatures, 199
    overuse syndrome, 132
    physician examination, 24
    swimming as rehabilitation medium, 189
    tennis, 166-167
    vicious cycle of inflexibility (VCIF), 180

Inner-Thigh Conditioner stretch, 127-129
Inner-Thigh Straddle stretch (runners), 184

J - K

joints, 23, 38-40, 304
    bursitis, 38-40
    cartilage, 38-40
    example of walking process, 38-40
    moveable, 38-40
    range of motion, 38-40, 304
    synovial fluid, 38-40

Knee Bender stretch (nighttime), 101
Knee-Neck stretch (pregnancy), 213
Kneeling Shin stretch (runners), 186
knees
    and hip flexibility, 30
    flexibility
        limited, 12
        testing, 11-12
        troubleshooting, 49
    stretches
        Diamond stretch, 104-105
        Knee Bender, 101
        Two Knees to the Chin stretch, 56
        Two Knees to the Side stretch, 56

L

Landing Eagle stretch, 66
Landing Gear Neck stretch (airplanes), 142
Landing Gear Up stretch (airplanes), 146-147
"Leaning Tower of Pisa" posture, 9-10
Leg Lifter, Two-Step stretch (nighttime), 102
Leg stretch (office), 119

legs
    femur bone, 185
    injuries
        ankles, 179
        hip flexor, 179
        hip joints, 179
        knees, 179
    physical labor stretches
        Hamstring Conditioner stretch, 126
        Inner-Thigh Conditioner stretch, 127-129
        Lower Body Standing stretch, 125
        One-Armer stretch, 129
        Standing Quad Conditioner stretch, 127
    pinching sensation, 274
    stretches
        Accelerator stretch, 151
        Birdie Hip stretch, 158
        Calves Pole stretch, 180
        Cart Quad stretch, 157
        Dynamic Quad stretch, 183
        Eagle Inner-Thigh stretch, 159
        En Garde lunges, 237
        Fighter Pilot stretch, 141
        Frog Squat stretch, 75
        Frog stretch, 196
        Front Hip Flexor stretch, 77
        Front Squat stretch, 74
        Hamstring Bench stretch, 174
        Hamstring stretch, 216
        Hamstring Striding stretch, 182
        Inner-Thigh Straddle stretch, 184
        Kneeling Shin stretch, 186
        Landing Eagle stretch, 66
        Leg Lifter, Two-Step stretch, 102
        One-Legged Climber stretch, 187
        Quad stretch, 203
        Shin Splits stretch, 195
        Shock Absorber stretch, 202

Side Quad stretch, 103
Sliding stretch, 175-176
Squat lunge, 76
Standing Calf stretch, 77
Standing Quad stretch, 173
Top of the Run stretch, 206
stretching
    importance of, 177-178
    misconceptions, 178
Level 1 Hamstring stretch, 268
Level 2 Hamstring stretch, 269
Level 3 Hamstring stretch, 270
lifestyles
    leisure activities
        aerobic sports, 27
        couch potatoes, 29
        endurance sports, 26-27
        Weekend Warriors, 28
    sitters, effect on muscles, 22
    standers, effect on muscles, 23
ligaments, 23, 304
    strains, rehabilitating, 24
limited flexibility in knees, 12
locked hips, 232
Long Driver Shoulder stretch (golf), 160-161
Lower Body Standing stretch (physical labor), 125
Lumbar Roll (driving), 150

M

Marathon Runners, flexibility, 25
mirrors, posture examination, 6-11
mixing stretching with other exercise programs, 46-47
Modified Pretzel stretch (hips), 257
mogul skiing, 203
Morning Hamstring stretch, 54-55
morning stretches
    Cat and Dog stretch, 58-59
    Hamstring stretch, 54-55
    Praying stretch, 59
    Torso Press-Up stretch, 60

Two Knees to the Chin stretch, 56
Two Knees to the Side stretch, 56
Undercover Body stretch, 54
Walking Wake-Up stretch, 61-62
moveable joints
    ball and socket, 38-40
    gliding, 38-40
    hinge, 38-40
    pivot joints, 38-40
muscles, 22
    aching, 22
    body awareness, 198
    bouncing during stretches, 182
    cold temperatures, proper warm-up, 199
    fascicles, 36-37
    fatigue, 23, 27
    flexibility
        adults versus children, 40
        specialists, searching, 31
    getting out of bed, 57
    inactivity, 41
    injuries, physician examination, 24
    neck toning, 63
    overused biceps, 129
    platysma, 62
    quadriceps, 103
    relationships to bones, 34
    scar tissue, 24
    shortened, 22
    shortening, 37
    spasms, 24, 304
    spinal erectors, 276
    strains, 22, 304
        rehabilitating, 24
    swimming, coordination of, 190
    tendon attachments, 37
    tendons, 24
    tennis
        injuries, 166-167
        movements, 165-166
    tension, 25
    tightness in pubescent children, 220
    types
        heart, 36-37
        skeletal, 36-37

smooth, 36-37
vacationing, compensating for, 40-41
"water ballet of the joints" (swimming), 190
weak triceps, 129
work process, 37
myofibrils, 36-37

N

Neck Toner stretch, 63
Neck Side-to-Side stretch, 286
Neck stretch (children), 230
necks
    cracking, 18
    flexibility, testing, 18
    indication of pain, 29
    pains, treating, 29
    stretches
        Back Neck stretch, 288
        Chin-Ups stretch, 289
        Ear to Shoulder stretch, 88
        Head Forward and Back stretch, 87
        Head Rotation stretch, 89
        Knee-Neck stretch, 213
        Landing Gear Neck stretch, 142
        Neck Side-to-Side stretch, 286
        Rotating Neck stretch, 113-114
        Seated Neck stretch, 287
        Tension Deleter stretch, 112
nighttime stretches
    Back Rockers stretch, 95
    benefits, 91-92
    Curtain Call stretch, 107
    Diamond stretch, 104-105
    Extended Back stretcher, 92-95
    Extended Side-to-Side stretch, 94
    Gentle Back stretch, 105
    guidelines, 91-92
    Knee Bender stretch, 101
    Leg Lifter stretch, 102
    One-Arm Twist stretch, 98-99

Rotating Rhythm stretch, 106
Seated Back stretch, 99
Seated Shoulder stretch, 96
Side Quad stretch, 103
Sitting Twist stretch, 100
Togetherness Side-to-Side stretch, 97
with partners, 91-92

O

oblique muscles, 66
office stretches
    Hamstring Standing stretch 120-121
    leg stretch, 119
    Programmer 1 stretch, 121
    Programmer 2 stretch, 122
    Quad Muscle Wake-Up stretch, 118
    Rotating Neck stretch, 113-114
    Sitting Hip stretch, 116
    Sitting Outside Hip stretch, 117
    Tension Deleter stretch, 112
One-Arm Seat stretch (driving), 150
One Knee Over stretch (back), 281
One Knee to Chest stretch (back), 275
One-Arm Twist stretch (nighttime), 98-99
One-Armer stretch (physical labor), 129
One-Foot stretch (children), 222
One-Legged Climber stretch (runners), 187
One-Legged Frog stretch (thighs), 264
Osgood-Slaghter disease (children), 219-220
Over Grip Net stretch (tennis), 169
Overhead Shrug stretch, 85
Overhead Side stretch (senior citizens), 234
overstretching during pregnancy, 210

overuse syndrome, 132, 304
overused biceps, 129

P

pain
    flexibility specialists, searching, 31
    sitting position, 30
    standing position, 30
    treating (necks), 29
parental supervision of children, 227
Partner Hip stretch (pregnancy), 218
Partner Side stretch (pregnancy), 217
pelvis (bones), 34
physical labor
    arthritis complaints, 124-125
    effects on
        back, 125
        hips, 125
        shoulders, 125
    lifters, 125
    repetitive motions, 124-125
    stretches, 124-125
        Backward Arm Conditioner stretch, 131-132
        Double-Handed stretch, 130
        Hamstring Conditioner stretch, 126
        Inner-Thigh Conditioner stretch, 127-129
        Lower Body Standing stretch, 125
        One-Armer stretch, 129
        Standing Quad Conditioner stretch, 127
    versus professional athletes, 124-125
    workers' compensation claims, 125
"pigeon-toed" (footstep patterns)
    causes, 5
    in athletes, 5
    straightening, 5
Pipe Bender stretch (work sites), 136

Pipe Twister stretch (work sites), 138
pivot joints, 38-40
platysma muscle, 62
Pointed Elbow stretch, 297
postures
    examining, 6-11
    side view, 10-11
    types
        "Leaning Tower of Pisa," 9-10
        "Statue of Liberty," 6
Praying stretch, 59
pregnancy
    overstretching, 210
    Relaxin hormone, 210
    stretches
        Back Bend Over stretch, 210
        Crossover stretch, 212
        Hamstring stretch, 216
        Knee-Neck stretch, 213
        Partner Hip stretch, 218
        Partner Side stretch, 217
        Side Quad stretch, 214
        Standing Shoulder Twist stretch, 211
        Two-Legged Pelvic Raise stretch, 215
    stretching
        dizziness, 212
        guidelines, 210
professional athletes
    effects of stretching, 43-45
    importance of flexibility, 44-45
    Price, Nick (golf), 44-45
Programmer stretch 1 (office), 121
Programmer stretch 2 (office), 122
puberty, effects, 220
Pushing Wrist stretch, 300

Q - R

Quad Muscle Wake-Up stretch (office), 118
Quad stretch (skiing), 203

quadriceps, 103, 304
  stretches
    Advanced Triangle Quad
      stretch, 266
    Chair lunge, 267

range of motion, 38, 304
rebuilding energy through
  stretches, 74
rehabilitating
  bone fractures, 23
  injuries through swimming,
    189
  ligament strains, 24
  muscle strains, 24
Relaxin hormone (pregnancy),
  210
retoning sitting muscles, 116
rollerbladers
  injuries
    hip joints, 179
    muscle fatigue, 179
  stretches
    One-Legged Climber
      stretch, 187
Rotating Neck stretch (office),
  113-114
Rotating Rhythm stretch
  (nighttime), 106
rotational flexibility, 304
  in golf, 155-156
runners
  injuries
    ankles, 179
    hip joints, 179
    knees, 179
  legs and stretching regimen,
    177-178
  stretches
    Calves Pole stretch, 180
    Dynamic Quad stretch,
      183
    Hamstring Striding
      stretch, 182
    Inner-Thigh Straddle
      stretch, 184
    Kneeling Shin stretch,
      186
    One-Legged Climber
      stretch, 187
    Shin Splint stretch, 250
    Standing Hip stretch, 185

S

S-shape (spinal column), 304
scar tissue, 304
  muscles, 24
searching for flexibility
  specialists, 31
Seated Back stretcher (nighttime), 99
Seated Hip stretch, 260
Seated Neck stretch, 287
Seated Rowing Motion
  stretch, 84
Seated Shoulder stretch
  (nighttime), 96
senior citizens
  hip replacement surgery,
    240
  locked hips, 232
  stretches
    Cross-Body Arm stretch,
      236
    En Garde lunge, 237
    Overhead Side stretch,
      234
    Senior Hamstring stretch,
      238
    Senior Modified Pretzel
      stretch, 240
    Senior Side-Quad stretch,
      241
    Side lunge, 238
    Standing Shoulder
      Twist stretch, 235
  stretching
    benefits, 233
    doctor consultation, 233
Senior Modified Pretzel stretch
  (senior citizens), 240
Senior Side-Quad stretch
  (senior citizens), 241
Serving stretches (tennis),
  170-171
Serving Tray stretch (airplanes),
  144
Shin Splints, 304
  stretch (runners), 250
  stretch (swimming), 195
Shock Absorber stretch
  (skiing), 202
shortened muscles, 37

Shoulder Arm Across the Body
  stretch, 290
Shoulder Back Roll (back), 278
Shoulder Shrug stretch, 83
Shoulder Twist stretch, 86
shoulders
  flexibility
    testing, 14-16
    troubleshooting, 49
  stretches
    Biceps stretch, 290
    Horizontal Towel
      stretch, 70
    Landing Gear Up stretch,
      146
    Long Driver Shoulder
      stretch, 160-161
    One-Arm Twist stretch,
      98-99
    Overhead Shrug
      stretch, 85
    Seated Rowing Motion
      stretch, 84
    Seated Shoulder
      stretch, 96
    Serving-Tray, Shoulder-
      Blade stretch, 144
    Shoulder Shrug
      stretch, 83
    Shoulder Twist stretch, 86
    Shoulder Arm Across the
      Body stretch, 290
    Sleeper stretch, 193, 292
    Triceps stretch, 291
    Vertical Towel stretch, 71
  tightness, 14-16
Side Bend stretch, 78
Side lunges (senior citizens),
  238
Side Overhead Arch (back), 282
Side-Quad stretch
  nighttime, 103
  pregnancy, 214
Side stretch (children), 224
Side Wrist stretch, 301
sitters
  effect on muscles, 22
  muscles, aching, 22
Sitting Hip stretch (office), 116
Sitting Lower-Back stretch, 277
sitting muscles, retoning, 116
Sitting Outside Hip stretch
  (office), 117

Sitting Twist stretch (nighttime), 100
skeletal muscles, 36-37
skiing
  moguls, 203
  stretches
    Black Diamond stretch, 205
    Edge Sharpener stretch, 200-201
    Quad stretch, 203
    Shock Absorber stretch, 202
    Standing Hip stretch, 204
    Top of the Run stretch, 206
Sleeper stretch
  shoulders, 292
  swimming, 193
sleeping and neck pain, 29
Sliding stretch (tennis), 175
smooth muscles, 36-37
Soccer stretch (children), 223
spinal
  discs, 304
  erector muscles, 276
spine, components, 140
sports medicine specialists, searching, 31
spouse as stretch partner, 91-92
  importance of communication, 100
Squat and Sit stretch, 80
Squat lunge, 76
"squeaking wheel," 48-49
standers, effect on muscles, 23
Standing Calf stretch, 77, 246-247
Standing Heel and Calf stretch, 248
Standing-Hip stretch
  runners, 185
  skiing, 204
Standing Inner-Thigh stretch (hips), 262
Standing Quad Conditioner (physical labor), 127
Standing Quad stretch (tennis), 173
Standing Shoulder Twist
  pregnancy, 211
  senior citizens, 235

starting stretching routines, 45-46
"Statue of Liberty" posture, 6
Steering-Wheel Twist (driving), 147
Straight Elbow stretch, 296
straightening
  "pigeon-toed" walks, 5
  "waddling duck" walks, 5
strains, rehabilitating
  ligaments, 24
  muscles, 24
Stretch Hamstring stretch (senior citizens), 238
stretch receptors, 47-48
stretches
  15-second hold, 47-48
  airplanes
    Banking Rotation stretch, 142
    comfort guidelines, 140
    Fighter Pilot stretch, 141
    Flaps-Up Arm stretch, 141
    guidelines, 140
    Landing Gear Neck stretch, 142
    Landing Gear Up stretch, 146
    Serving-Tray, Shoulder-Blade stretch, 144
    Tail-Section stretch, 144
  ankles, 172, 251
  back
    One Knee Over stretch, 281
    One Knee to Chest stretch, 275
    Shoulder Back Roll stretch, 278
    Side Overhead Arch stretch, 282
    Sitting Lower-Back stretch, 277
    Torso stretch, 279
    Two Knees Over stretch, 280
    Two Knees to Chest stretch, 276
    Bend Over Twist stretch, 66
    benefits in golf swing, 156-157

Both Sides Body Conditioner stretch, 134
calves
  Pole stretch, 180
  Standing Calf stretch, 246-247
  Standing Heel and Calf stretch, 248
carpal tunnel syndrome
  Backhand Push stretch, 114
  Wrist Relievers, 115-116
children
  Back Leaner stretch, 226
  Campfire Sitting stretch, 228
  Cannon Ball stretch, 225
  Hamstring stretch, 227
  Hands Above the Head stretch, 222
  Neck Stretch, 230
  One-Foot stretch, 222
  Side stretch, 224
  Soccer stretch, 223
  Swordsmen lunge, 229-230
driving, 147
  Accelerator stretch, 151
  Door stretch, 148
  Head-Rest Arm stretch, 149
  Lumbar Roll, 150
  One-Arm Seat stretch, 150
  Steering-Wheel Twist, 147
Ear to Shoulder, 88
elbows
  Pointed Elbow stretch, 297
  Straight Elbow stretch, 296
  Table Elbow stretch, 297
  Tennis Elbow stretch, 299
  Wrist Twist Stretch Down, 298
energy
  Frog Squat stretch, 75
  Front Hip Flexor stretch, 77-78
  Front Squat stretch, 74-75
  Hands Up stretch, 78
  rebuilding, 74

Side Bend stretch, 78
Squat and Sit stretch, 80
Squat lunge, 76
Standing Calf stretch, 77
feet, 252
Ankle Rotation stretch, 253
Front Bend, 64
gardeners
Back Planter stretch, 132
Hamstring Planter stretch, 134-136
golf
Birdie Hip stretch, 158
Cart Quad stretch, 157
Eagle Inner Thigh stretch, 159
Long Driver Shoulder stretch, 160-161
hamstrings
Butterfly stretch, 271
Level 1 Hamstring stretch, 268
Level 2 Hamstring stretch, 269
Level 3 Hamstring stretch, 270
Head Forward and Back stretch, 87
Head Rotation stretch, 89
hips
Full Pretzel stretch, 258
Modified Pretzel stretch, 257
Seated Hip stretch, 260
Standing Inner-Thigh stretch, 262
Horizontal Towel stretch, 70
Landing Eagle stretch, 66
morning
Cat and Dog stretch, 58-59
Hamstring stretch, 54-55
Praying stretch, 59
Torso Press-Up stretch, 60
Two Knees to the Chin stretch, 56
Two Knees to the Side stretch, 56
Undercover Body stretch, 54
Walking Wake-Up stretch, 61-62

neck
Back Neck stretch, 288
Chin-Ups stretch, 289
Neck Side-to-Side stretch, 286
Neck Toner stretch, 62
Seated Neck stretch, 287
nighttime
Back Rockers stretch, 95
Curtain Call stretch, 107
Diamond stretch, 104-105
Extended Back stretcher, 92-95
Extended Side-to-Side stretch, 94
Gentle Back stretch, 105
Knee Bender stretch, 101
Leg Lifter stretch, 102
One-Arm Twist stretch, 98-99
Rotating Rhythm stretch, 106
Seated Back stretch, 99
Seated Shoulder stretch, 96
Side Quad stretch, 103
Sitting Twist stretch, 100
Togetherness Side-to-Side stretch, 97
office
Hamstring Standing stretch, 120-121
Leg stretch, 119
Programmer stretch 1, 121
Programmer stretch 2, 122
Quad Muscle Wake-Up stretch, 118
Rotating Neck stretch, 113-114
Sitting Hip stretch, 116
Sitting Outside Hip stretch, 117
Tension Deleter stretch, 112
physical labor
Backward Arm Conditioner stretch, 131-132
Double-Handed stretch, 130

Hamstring Conditioner stretch, 126
Inner-Thigh Conditioner stretch, 127-129
Lower Body Standing stretch, 125
One-Armer stretch, 129
Standing Quad Conditioner stretch, 127
post-skiing regimen, 204
pregnancy
Back Bend Over stretch, 210
Crossover stretch, 212
Hamstring stretch, 216
Knee-Neck stretch, 213
Partner Hip stretch, 218
Partner Side stretch, 217
Side Quad stretch, 214
Standing Shoulder Twist stretch, 211
Two-Legged Pelvic Raise stretch, 215
quadriceps
Advanced Triangle Quad stretch, 266
Chair lunge, 267
runners
Calves Pole stretch, 180
Dynamic Quad stretch, 183
Hamstring Striding stretch, 182
Inner-Thigh Straddle stretch, 184
Kneeling Shin stretch, 186
One-Legged Climber stretch, 187
Shin Splint stretch, 250
Standing Hip stretch, 185
senior citizens
Cross-Body Arm stretch, 236-237
En Garde lunge, 237
Overhead Side stretch, 234
Senior Hamstring stretch, 238
Senior Modified Pretzel stretch, 240
Senior Side-Quad stretch, 241

Side lunge, 238
Standing Shoulder Twist
stretch, 235
shoulders
Biceps stretch, 290
Shoulder Arm Across the
Body stretch, 290
Sleeper stretch, 292
Triceps, 291
sitting muscles, retoning,
116
skiing
Black Diamond stretch,
205
Edge Sharpener stretch,
200-201
Quad stretch, 203
Shock Absorber stretch,
202
Standing-Hip stretch, 204
Top of the Run stretch,
206
swimming
Freestyle stretch, 194
Frog stretch, 196
Shin Splits stretch, 195
Sleeper stretch, 193
tennis
Ankle stretcher, 172
Back Racket stretch, 167
Biceps Fence stretch,
171-172
First Serve stretch, 170
Hamstring Bench stretch,
174
Over Grip Net stretch,
169
serving overview,
170-171
Sliding stretch, 175
Standing Quad stretch,
173
Under Grip Net stretch,
168
tension relief, 82-86
Overhead Shrug stretch,
85
Seated Rowing Motion
stretch, 84
Shoulder Shrug stretch, 83
Shoulder Twist stretch, 86

thighs
Frog stretch, 263
One-Legged Frog stretch,
264
toes, 252
towel-free, 69
Vertical Towel stretch, 71
Wall Side Bend stretch, 68
with partners, 91-92
importance of communi-
cation, 100
work site
Pipe Bender stretch, 136
Pipe Twister stretch, 138
wrists
Pushing Wrist stretch,
300
Side Wrists stretch, 301
stretching
Achilles tendon, 180
ankles, troubleshooting, 49
bouncing effects, 182
animal instincts, 58, 178
back, doctor consultation,
273-274
bridge of energy, 74
children
encouraging daily
regimen, 220
parental communication,
227
effects on pro athletes,
43-45
guidelines, 47
inactive muscles, 41
legs
importance of, 177-178
misconceptions, 178
out of balance body, 48-49
pregnancy
dizziness, 212
guidelines, 210
record breaking perfor-
mances, 199
senior citizens, benefits, 233
"squeaking wheel," 48-49
starting point, launching,
45-46
stretch receptors, 47-48
using with other exercise
programs, 46-47
vicious cycle of inflexibility
(VCIF), 180

stretching balance, 48, 304
Supermodel body type, 26
swimming
injury rehabilitation, 189
muscle coordination, 190
myths on stretching, 193
shoulder resistance, 193
stretches
Freestyle stretch, 194
Fog stretch, 196
Shin Splits stretch, 195
Sleeper stretch, 193
"water ballet of the joints,"
190-192
Swordsmen lunge (children),
229-230
synovial fluid (joints), 38-40

T

Table Elbow stretch, 297
Tail-Section stretch (airplanes),
144
tandem stretches, 92
teaching children stretching
techniques, 220
tendons, 24, 304
muscle attachments, 37
tennis
elbow, 166-167, 304
injury potential, 166-167
muscle movement, 165-166
stretches
Ankle stretch, 172
Back Racket stretch, 167
Biceps Fence stretcher,
171-172
Elbow stretch, 299
First Serve stretch, 170
Hamstring Bench stretch,
174
Over Grip Net stretch,
169
serving overview,
170-171
Sliding stretch, 175
Standing Quad stretch,
173
Under Grip Net stretch,
168

tension
  effects on body, 82
  relaxer stretches
    Overhead Shrug
      stretch, 85
    Seated Rowing Motion
      stretch, 84
    Shoulder Shrug
      stretch, 83
    Shoulder Twist stretch, 86
  stretches
    Curtain Call stretch, 107
    Rotating Rhythm stretch,
      106
Tension Deleter stretch
  (office), 112
testing flexibility
  ankles, 13
  elbows, 16
  hips, 13-14
  knees, 11-12
  neck, 18
  shoulders, 14-16
  wrists, 17
thigh stretches
  Frog stretch, 263
  One-Legged Frog stretch,
    264
tibias (bones), 34
toe stretches, 252
Togetherness Side-to-Side
  stretch (nighttime), 97
toning facial muscles, 62-63
Top of the Run stretch (skiing),
  206
torso stretches
  Banking Rotation stretch,
    142
  Crossover stretch, 212
  Door stretch, 148
  Freestyle stretch, 194
  Overhead Side stretch, 234
  Partner Side stretch, 217
  Senior Hamstring stretch,
    238
  Senior Side Quad stretch,
    241
  Side Bend stretch, 78
  Side lunge, 238
  Standing Shoulder Twist
    stretch, 211
  Torso Back stretch, 279
  Two-Legged Pelvic Raise
    stretch, 215
torso muscles, 56
Torso Press-Up stretch, 60
towel-free stretches, 69
treating
  backaches, 30
  neck pains, 29
Triceps stretch (shoulders), 291
troubleshooting flexibility, 49
Two Knees Over stretch
  (back), 280
Two Knees to Chest stretch
  (back), 276
Two Knees to the Chin
  stretch, 56
Two Knees to the Side
  stretch, 56
Two-Legged Pelvic Raise stretch
  (pregnancy), 215

U - V

Under Grip Net stretch (ten-
  nis), 168
Undercover Body stretch, 54
upper-body stretches
  Programmer 1, 121
  Programmer 2, 122

vacationing muscles, compensating for, 40-41
vertebrae, 140
Vertical Towel stretch, 71
vicious cycle of inflexibility
  (VCIF), 180, 304

W - Z

"waddling duck" (footstep
  patterns)
    causes, 5
    straightening, 5
waking up, blood pressure, 59
walking and joint movement,
  38-40
Walking Wake-Up stretch,
  61-62
Wall Side Bend stretch, 68
warming up muscles in cold
  temperatures, 199
"water ballet of the joints"
  (swimming), 190-192
weak triceps, 129
work-site stretches
  Pipe Bender stretch, 136
  Pipe Twister stretch, 138
Workout Woman (body types),
  25-26
Wrist Twist Stretch Down, 298
wrists
  carpal tunnel syndrome
    Backhand Push stretch,
      114
    Wrist Relievers, 115-116
  flexibility, testing, 17
  stretches
    Over Grip Net stretch,
      169
    Pushing Wrist stretch,
      300
    Side Wrist stretch, 301
    Under Grip Net stretch,
      168
    Wrist Twist Stretch
      Down, 298